STROKE HOME CARE GUIDE

FOR PATIENTS AND CAREGIVERS

Dr. A. MITRA, MBBS, MD, DMI.

Disclaimer:

The information provided in this book is intended for educational purposes only. While every effort has been made to ensure accuracy and relevance, readers are advised to consult healthcare professionals for personalized advice and treatment options tailored to individual circumstances. The author and publisher disclaim any liability arising directly or indirectly from the use or application of the contents of this book.

DEDICATION

To all the resilient stroke survivors and their dedicated caregivers, whose unwavering strength and compassion inspire us every day. This guide is a testament to your courage, a resource crafted with your unique journeys in mind. May it provide support, knowledge, and hope as you navigate the path to recovery together.

CONTENTS

ACKNOWLEDGMENTS

I am deeply grateful to everyone who contributed to the creation of the "Stroke Home Care Guide." Special thanks to the patients and caregivers for sharing their experiences, and to the medical professionals whose expertise shaped the guide. My family and friends' unwavering support has been a driving force, and I also appreciate my editor and publisher for their dedication in bringing this book to life. Thank you all for making this endeavor possible.

1. UNDERSTANDING STROKE

What is a Stroke?

Imagine your brain is a city, and blood is like the trucks that deliver food and supplies. A stroke happens when one of those delivery trucks gets stuck or has an accident. It cannot get the important things your brain needs to different areas, and those parts of the brain might get weak or damaged.

There are two main types of strokes:

- **Blocked Stroke:** This is like a traffic jam in the city. A blood clot blocks the path, stopping the delivery truck from reaching its destination.
- **Bleeding Stroke:** This is like a burst pipe in the city. A blood vessel breaks, causing flooding and damaging the surrounding areas.

A stroke can happen to anyone, at any age. But there are things you can do to lower your chances of getting one, and things you can do to help someone if they have a stroke. We will learn more about those later.

Here are some of the signs that someone might be having a stroke:

- Sudden numbness or weakness in the face, arm, or leg (often on one side only)
- Trouble speaking or understanding words
- Confusion
- Problems seeing in one or both eyes
- Dizziness or trouble walking

If you think someone might be having a stroke, remember the acronym FAST:

- **F**ace drooping
- **A**rm weakness
- **S**peech difficulty
- **T**ime to call emergency services.

The faster you get help, the better the chances of a full recovery.

Types of Strokes

Remember how we learned about strokes being like traffic trouble in the brain city? In previous section, we talked about the big picture. Now, let us zoom in and see the two main types of traffic jams that can cause strokes:

1. Blocked Stroke: The Traffic Jam Caused by a Clot

Imagine a big, bad blood clot is like a grumpy truck driver who parked his vehicle right in the middle of a busy street. This blocks other trucks from delivering their supplies, just like the clot blocks blood flow to parts of the brain. Here is how it happens:

- **Sticky Situation:** Sometimes, fatty substances like cholesterol can build up in the blood vessels, making them narrow and sticky.
- **Clot Formation:** These sticky spots can trap blood cells, forming a clot that blocks the flow.
- **Brain in Trouble:** With the blood flow blocked, the brain cells beyond the clot do not get the oxygen and nutrients they need, and they start to die. This can cause weakness, numbness, or even trouble speaking, depending on which part of the brain is affected.

2. Bleeding Stroke: The Burst Pipe Causing Chaos

Think of a burst pipe in the city. It is like a weak blood vessel in the brain that suddenly breaks. This causes bleeding in the brain, damaging the surrounding areas. Here is what happens:

- **Weak Walls:** High blood pressure or other health problems can weaken the walls of blood vessels in the brain.
- **The Big Burst:** If the pressure gets too high, the weakened vessel cannot hold back and bursts, causing bleeding.
- **Brain Damage:** The bleeding puts pressure on and damages the brain tissue around it. This can lead to similar problems as a blocked stroke, like weakness, confusion, or vision problems.

Which One is Worse?

Both types of strokes are serious and need immediate medical attention. It is important to get help quickly so doctors can treat the stroke and minimize the damage. They can use different methods depending on the type of stroke.

Remember: Even though there are two main types, strokes can be different for everyone. The important thing is to know the FAST signs and call for help immediately if you suspect a stroke.

Signs and Symptoms of Stroke

Imagine your brain is a giant control center for your body. A stroke happens when something goes wrong with the blood flow to this center, causing problems with different parts of the body. But how do you know if someone is having a stroke? Here, we will learn the **FAST** signs – a simple way to remember the key symptoms:

F - Face Drooping: Does one side of the face look different? Is there a droop in one eye or corner of the mouth? This could be a sign that the muscles in the face are not working properly.

A - Arm Weakness: Can the person raise both arms equally? Does one arm feel weak or numb? This weakness can happen on one side of the body, depending on which part of the brain is affected.

S - Speech Difficulty: Is the person slurring their words? Are they having trouble understanding what you are saying? Speech problems can occur when the areas of the brain responsible for language are affected by a stroke.

T - Time to Call Emergency Services.

These signs can appear suddenly, so it is crucial to act FAST. Every minute counts when someone is having a stroke. The sooner they get medical attention, the better the chance of recovery. Here are some other signs to look out for, even if they do not perfectly match FAST:

- **Sudden Confusion:** Does the person seem confused or disoriented? This can happen if the part of the brain responsible for thinking is affected.
- **Vision Problems:** Is the person having trouble seeing in one or both eyes? This could be a sign that the blood flow to the area of the brain responsible for vision is blocked.
- **Dizziness or Trouble Walking:** Does the person feel dizzy or unsteady on their feet? This can be caused by problems with balance and coordination due to the stroke.

Remember: Do not wait to see if the symptoms go away. Even if they seem mild, call emergency services immediately. The quicker someone gets help, the less damage the stroke can cause. By learning the FAST signs and taking action quickly, you can help someone having a stroke get the treatment they need.

Risk Factors for Stroke

We learned about the different types of strokes and how to recognize them earlier. Now, let us talk about things that can increase your chances of having a stroke, like hazards on a highway for your brain. These are called risk factors, and the good news is there are ways to manage them.

Think of your brain like a city with blood vessels as highways. Here are some risk factors that can cause problems on these highways:

- **High Blood Pressure:** This is like having too much traffic on the road. The constant pressure can damage the blood vessels and make them more likely to burst or narrow.
- **High Cholesterol:** This is like sticky gunk building up on the highways, making them narrower and easier to clog with debris.
- **Diabetes:** This can damage blood vessels and make them more likely to burst or become blocked.
- **Smoking:** Smoking is like a polluter on the highway, damaging the blood vessels and making them more likely to get clogged.
- **Obesity:** Being overweight puts extra strain on your heart, which can lead to high blood pressure and other problems that increase stroke risk.
- **Inactivity:** Not exercising regularly can contribute to other risk factors like high blood pressure and cholesterol.
- **Unhealthy Diet:** Eating too much unhealthy food like processed meats, sugary drinks, and unhealthy fats can worsen other risk factors.
- **Sleep Apnea:** This is a condition where you stop breathing for short periods during sleep. It can increase blood pressure and stress on the heart, raising stroke risk.
- **Atrial Fibrillation:** This is an irregular heartbeat that can lead to blood clots forming in the heart and traveling to the brain, causing a stroke.
- **Family History:** If someone close in your family has had a stroke, you may be at a slightly higher risk.

The good news is, you can take action to control many of these risk factors. Here are some sways to keep your brain's highways healthy:

- **Eat a healthy diet:** Eat plenty of fruits, vegetables, and whole grains. Limit processed foods, sugary drinks, and unhealthy fats.

- **Exercise regularly:** Aim for at least 30 minutes of moderate-intensity exercise most days of the week.
- **Maintain a healthy weight:** Talk to your doctor about a healthy weight goal for you.
- **Manage stress:** Find healthy ways to manage stress, like yoga, meditation, or spending time in nature.
- **Control your blood pressure and cholesterol:** Work with your doctor to manage these through medication, lifestyle changes, or both.
- **Quit smoking:** Smoking is one of the most significant risk factors for stroke. There are many resources available to help you quit.
- **Get enough sleep:** Aim for 7-8 hours of quality sleep each night.
- **Talk to your doctor about sleep apnea and atrial fibrillation:** If you suspect you might have either of these conditions, get checked by your doctor.
- **See your doctor regularly:** Get regular checkups and screenings for risk factors like high blood pressure and cholesterol.

Remember: By taking control of these risk factors, you can significantly reduce your chances of having a stroke. Talk to your doctor about your individual risk factors and create a plan to keep your brain healthy.

Preventing Stroke

In the last chapter, we learned about the things that can increase your risk of having a stroke, like traffic jams on the highways of your brain. The good news is, there are many things you can do to prevent strokes and keep those highways running smoothly. Think of it like putting up road signs and taking care of your car to avoid accidents. Here are some key ways to prevent stroke:

1. Manage Your Blood Pressure:

- Imagine high blood pressure is like having way too many cars on the road at once. This constant pressure can damage the blood vessels and make them more likely to burst or narrow.
- **The Fix:** Regularly check your blood pressure at home or with your doctor. If it is high, follow your doctor's advice on medication, healthy eating, and exercise to lower it.

2. Control Your Cholesterol:

- Think of cholesterol as sticky gunk building up on the highways, making them narrower and easier to clog with debris. This can block the flow of blood to your brain.
- **The Fix:** Eat a healthy diet low in saturated and trans fats, found in processed foods and fried items. Choose healthy fats like those found in fish, nuts, and avocadoes. Exercise regularly to help your body manage cholesterol levels.

3. Maintain a Healthy Diet:

- Your brain needs the right fuel just like a car needs the right gas. Eating a healthy diet is crucial for keeping your blood pressure, cholesterol, and weight in check.
- **The Fix:** Fill your plate with fruits, vegetables, and whole grains. Choose lean protein sources like fish, chicken, and beans. Limit sugary drinks, processed foods, and unhealthy fats.

4. Exercise Regularly:

- Just like a car needs regular maintenance, your body needs exercise to stay healthy. Exercise helps control blood pressure, cholesterol, and weight, all of which are risk factors for stroke.

- **The Fix:** Aim for at least 30 minutes of moderate-intensity exercise most days of the week. Brisk walking, swimming, or biking are all great options.

5. Manage Stress:

- Chronic stress can put extra strain on your heart and blood vessels, increasing your risk of stroke.
- **The Fix:** Find healthy ways to manage stress, like yoga, meditation, or spending time in nature. Talking to friends and family or a therapist can also be helpful.

6. Quit Smoking:

- Smoking is one of the biggest risk factors for stroke. It damages blood vessels and increases the risk of blood clots.
- **The Fix:** Quitting smoking is one of the best things you can do for your overall health, including your brain. There are many resources available to help you quit, like support groups and medication.

7. Get Enough Sleep:

- Just like a car needs time to rest and refuel, your body needs enough sleep to function properly. Sleep deprivation can contribute to high blood pressure and other risk factors for stroke.
- **The Fix:** Aim for 7-8 hours of quality sleep each night. Establish a regular sleep schedule and create a relaxing bedtime routine.

8. Talk to Your Doctor:

- They can check you for risk factors like high blood pressure, diabetes, and sleep apnea. Early detection and treatment can significantly reduce your risk of stroke.

- **The Fix:** Schedule regular checkups with your doctor. Discuss your risk factors and create a personalized prevention plan together.

9. Know the Warning Signs of Stroke:

- Being aware of the FAST signs (Face drooping, Arm weakness, Speech difficulty, Time to call emergency services) can help you recognize a stroke in yourself or someone else and get immediate medical attention. Early treatment can minimize brain damage and improve recovery.

10. Live a Healthy Lifestyle:

- All the tips above add up to a healthy lifestyle that keeps your brain and body strong. Managing weight, avoiding excessive alcohol consumption, and maintaining good oral hygiene can also contribute to stroke prevention.

Remember: By following these tips and taking control of your health, you can significantly reduce your risk of stroke and keep your brain highways running smoothly for a long and healthy life.

The Role of Genetics in Stroke Risk

We have learned a lot about how to keep our brains healthy and prevent strokes. But did you know that your genes, the instruction manuals from your parents, can also play a role in stroke risk?

Think of your genes like blueprints for building your body. Some genes might make you taller, while others might influence your eye color. Genes can also affect your risk of certain diseases, including stroke.

Here are how genes might be involved in stroke risk:

- **Family History:** If someone close in your family, like a parent or sibling, has had a stroke, you might be at a slightly higher risk. This does not mean you will definitely have a stroke, but it is a good reason to be extra careful about managing other risk factors.
- **Genetic Variations:** Sometimes, there are tiny variations in your genes that can slightly increase your chances of developing certain health problems, including stroke. These variations might affect how your body processes cholesterol, blood pressure, or blood clotting.

Important things to remember about genes and stroke risk:

- **Not a Guarantee:** Having a family history or a specific gene variation does not mean you will for sure have a stroke. It is just one piece of the puzzle.
- **Focus on Controllable Factors:** While you cannot change your genes, you can control many other risk factors for stroke, like diet, exercise, and managing blood pressure. By focusing on these, you can significantly reduce your overall risk.
- **Limited Knowledge:** Scientists are still learning about the exact role of genes in stroke. There is likely a combination of genes and lifestyle factors at play.

What can you do?

- **Talk to your doctor:** If you have a family history of stroke, discuss your risk with your doctor. They can assess your overall health and recommend personalized strategies for prevention.
- **Maintain a healthy lifestyle:** Focus on controlling the risk factors you can manage, like diet, exercise, and stress. This is the best way to keep your brain healthy, regardless of your genes.
- **Stay informed:** Research on genetics and stroke is ongoing. Keep yourself updated on new information and advancements in the field.

Remember: Genetics might play a role, but it does not have to control your destiny. By understanding your risk factors and taking proactive steps, you can empower yourself to keep your brain healthy and reduce your risk of stroke.

2. COMING HOME AFTER STROKE

Safety at Home

Imagine your home as a nest for healing after a stroke. Just like a bird needs a safe and comfortable nest to recover from injury, a stroke survivor needs a home environment that supports their recovery journey. This chapter will guide you on transforming your home into a haven for healing and regaining independence.

Safety First:

- **Fall Prevention:** Falls are a major concern after a stroke. Identify and remove tripping hazards like loose rugs, clutter, and uneven flooring. Install grab bars in bathrooms and near stairs. Ensure good lighting throughout the house to improve visibility.
- **Assistive Devices:** Consider the needs of the stroke survivor. Grab bars, shower chairs, raised toilet seats, and handrails can provide extra support and stability. Elevated toilet seats and specialized utensils can make daily routines easier.
- **Electrical Safety:** Address potential electrical hazards by covering unused outlets and ensuring cords are tucked away to prevent tripping.

Accessibility for All:

- **Clear Pathways:** Ensure wide, clear pathways throughout the house to allow easy movement with walkers, wheelchairs, or braces. Rearrange furniture if necessary to create enough space for maneuvering.
- **Doorways:** Widen doorways if needed to accommodate wheelchairs or assistive devices. Consider installing automatic door openers for easier access.

- **Lower Cabinets:** Make frequently used items in the kitchen and bathroom easily accessible by relocating them to lower cabinets or shelves.

Living Room Adjustments:

- **Comfortable Seating:** Choose firm and supportive chairs with armrests to help with standing and sitting.
- **Lighting:** Ensure good lighting throughout the room to avoid shadows and improve visibility.
- **Communication Tools:** If the stroke survivor has difficulty speaking, consider having picture boards or communication aids readily available.

Bathroom Safety:

- **Shower Chair and Grab Bars:** Install a shower chair with a back and armrests for stability during showering. Grab bars should be placed near the toilet, tub, and shower for added support.
- **Non-Slip Mats:** Use non-slip mats in the bathtub and shower to prevent falls.

Kitchen Adjustments:

- **Clear Countertops:** Keep frequently used items within easy reach on lower countertops. Declutter to avoid creating obstacles.
- **Sharp Objects:** Store sharp knives and other utensils safely out of reach.
- **Adaptive Tools:** Consider adaptive cooking tools like one-handed openers or rocker knives to make meal preparation easier.

Remember: Every stroke survivor is unique, so personalize these adjustments to their specific needs and limitations. Here are some additional tips:

- **Involve the Stroke Survivor:** When possible, involve the stroke survivor in the planning process. Their input on what feels comfortable and safe is crucial.
- **Start Small:** Do not try to do everything at once. Make gradual changes over time to avoid overwhelming yourself or the stroke survivor.
- **Seek Professional Help:** Occupational therapists can assess the home and recommend specific modifications to optimize safety and accessibility.

By creating a safe and supportive home environment, you can significantly contribute to the stroke survivor's recovery and well-being. Imagine the joy of seeing them regain independence and navigate their home with confidence – a true testament to the power of a well-prepared haven for healing.

Working with the Care Team

After a stroke, a whole team of people can come together to help your loved one recover. It is like having a superhero squad dedicated to their well-being. This chapter will introduce you to the key members of this care team and explain how you can work together for the best possible outcome.

The Superheroes of Stroke Care:

- **Doctor:** The doctor is like the team leader, overseeing the overall care plan. They will diagnose the type of stroke, prescribe medications, and monitor progress.
- **Nurse:** Nurses are your daily support system. They provide hands-on care, manage medications, and answer your questions.
- **Physical Therapist:** This superhero helps your loved one regain movement and strength. They teach exercises to improve mobility, coordination, and balance.

- **Occupational Therapist:** This therapist focuses on helping your loved one regain independence in daily activities like bathing, dressing, and eating. They can recommend adaptive equipment and modify tasks as needed.
- **Speech-Language Pathologist:** If your loved one has difficulty speaking or swallowing, this therapist will help them improve communication skills and relearn safe swallowing techniques.
- **Social Worker:** This superhero connects your family with resources and support services available in the community. They can also help with emotional adjustments and navigating social situations after a stroke.

Working Together for Success:

- **Communication is Key:** Open communication between you, the care team, and your loved one is crucial. Ask questions, express concerns, and share any observations you have about your loved one's progress.
- **Team Meetings:** Attend scheduled team meetings to discuss the care plan, ask questions, and provide updates on your loved one's progress at home.
- **Respecting Roles:** Each member of the care team has their expertise. Trust their recommendations and work together to achieve the best outcome.
- **Be an Advocate:** You are a vital part of your loved one's care team. Do not be afraid to ask questions, voice your concerns, and advocate for their needs.

Building a Strong Team:

- **Ask Questions:** When meeting each team member, understand their role and how they contribute to your loved one's care plan.

- **Do not Hesitate to Speak Up:** If you have any concerns or questions, do not hesitate to speak with any member of the care team.
- **Share Information:** Provide the team with relevant information about your loved one's medical history, daily routines, and any pre-existing conditions.

Remember: Working collaboratively with the stroke care team creates a strong support system for your loved one. By understanding each member's role and communicating effectively, you can empower the team to work together towards a successful recovery journey.

Understanding Medications

Imagine your body is a complex machine, and after a stroke, some parts might need a little extra help to work properly. Medications are like tools doctors use to fine-tune this machine and promote healing. This chapter will guide you through the world of medications commonly prescribed after a stroke, helping you understand their purpose and potential side effects.

The Essential Toolkit:

- **Blood Thinners:** These medications, like aspirin or blood thinners, help prevent blood clots from forming and causing another stroke. It is important to take them exactly as prescribed to avoid excessive bleeding.
- **Cholesterol-Lowering Medications:** These medications, like statins, help lower bad cholesterol levels in the blood, reducing the risk of future strokes.
- **Blood Pressure Medications:** Medications like ACE inhibitors or diuretics help control high blood pressure, a major risk factor for stroke. Consistent use is crucial for long-term management.

- **Anti-Seizure Medications:** If the stroke affects certain areas of the brain, there is a chance of seizures. These medications help prevent or control seizures.

Understanding Side Effects:

Every medication can have side effects, but some are more common than others. It is important to be aware of them and discuss them with your doctor. Here are some general possibilities:

- **Blood Thinners:** These can increase the risk of bleeding, so be cautious during activities that might cause cuts or bruises.
- **Cholesterol-Lowering Medications:** These may cause muscle aches or fatigue in some people.
- **Blood Pressure Medications:** Dizziness, headaches, or fatigue can be potential side effects.
- **Anti-Seizure Medications:** These can cause drowsiness, dizziness, or mood changes in some individuals.

Remember: Do not stop taking your medications or adjust the dosage without consulting your doctor.

Important Tips for Medication Management:

- **Keep a Medication List:** Maintain an updated list of all medications your loved one is taking, including dosages and prescribing doctors. This helps avoid confusion and ensures proper medication management.
- **Schedule Reminders:** Set reminders or use pill organizers to ensure medications are taken on time and in the correct dosages.
- **Ask Questions:** Do not hesitate to ask your doctor or pharmacist any questions you have about medications, side effects, or potential interactions with other medications or supplements.

- **Report Side Effects:** If you experience any concerning side effects, inform your doctor right away. They might adjust the medication or dosage.

Working with the Doctor:

- **Open Communication:** Maintain open communication with your doctor about any questions or concerns you have regarding medications.
- **Review Regularly:** Attend scheduled appointments for medication reviews. The doctor might adjust medications or dosages based on your loved one's progress and overall health.

By understanding medications and working collaboratively with the doctor, you can ensure your loved one receives the right treatment to promote healing and prevent future complications.

Managing Daily Activities

After a stroke, some everyday tasks might feel challenging. But just like learning a new skill, with practice and support, your loved one can regain independence in their daily activities. This chapter will guide you on ways to break down daily tasks, explore adaptive techniques, and empower your loved one to manage their routines with confidence.

Breaking Down the Tasks:

Imagine getting dressed in the morning. It might seem simple, but after a stroke, it could involve several steps like putting on socks, pants, shirts, and shoes. By breaking down this task into smaller, manageable steps, it becomes less overwhelming. Here are some tips for simplifying daily activities:

- **Focus on One Step at a Time:** Instead of trying to do everything at once, focus on completing one step of the task at a time. Celebrate small successes and gradually increase complexity.

- **Visual Aids:** Create visual aids like picture charts or checklists to remind your loved one of the steps involved in each activity.

Adaptive Techniques and Tools:

Sometimes, a little creativity and the right tools can make a big difference. Here are some examples of adaptive techniques and tools that can be helpful:

- **Dressing:** Button extenders, long-handled shoe horns, and dressing sticks can make getting dressed easier.
- **Bathing:** Shower chairs, grab bars, and hand-held showerheads can increase safety and independence in the bathroom.
- **Eating:** Weighted utensils, plates with raised edges, and spill-proof cups can make mealtimes less frustrating.
- **Reaching:** Grabbers can help retrieve objects from high shelves or off the floor.

Encouraging Independence:

- **Offer Choices:** Whenever possible, offer your loved one choices to maintain a sense of control. Let them choose which outfit to wear or what to eat for breakfast.
- **Positive Reinforcement:** Celebrate their successes, no matter how small. Encouragement and positive reinforcement can go a long way in boosting confidence and motivation.
- **Respect Their Pace:** Everyone recovers at their own pace. Avoid pushing your loved one too hard. Let them take their time and gradually increase their participation in daily tasks.

Occupational Therapy:

An occupational therapist can be a valuable resource. They can assess your loved one's needs, recommend adaptive techniques and tools, and teach them strategies for regaining independence in daily activities.

Remember: Regaining independence takes time and patience. By breaking down tasks, exploring adaptive techniques, and offering encouragement, you can empower your loved one to manage their daily routines with confidence and a renewed sense of accomplishment.

Managing Appointments and Follow-Up Care

After a stroke, regular doctor visits and therapy sessions become an important part of the recovery journey. Think of it like a car needing regular tune-ups to keep running smoothly. This chapter will guide you on managing appointments, understanding follow-up care plans, and ensuring your loved one receives the best possible care on their road to recovery.

Scheduling Appointments:

- **Keep a Calendar:** Maintain a dedicated calendar to track upcoming doctor appointments, therapy sessions, and any other important health-related events.
- **Reminders:** Set reminders on your phone or use a calendar app to ensure you do not miss any appointments.
- **Transportation:** Plan transportation to and from appointments in advance. Consider carpooling with family members or using public transportation options.

Preparing for Appointments:

- **Gather Information:** Before each appointment, gather any relevant information, such as a list of medications your loved one is taking or any recent symptoms they've been experiencing.
- **Write Down Questions:** Encourage your loved one to write down any questions they have for the doctor or therapist.

- **Bring Support:** Consider attending appointments with your loved one to take notes, ask clarifying questions, and provide any additional information needed.

Understanding Follow-Up Care Plans:

- **The Doctor's Roadmap:** The doctor will create a follow-up care plan outlining the recommended course of treatment, including medications, therapy sessions, and lifestyle modifications.
- **Importance of Follow-Up:** Regular follow-up appointments allow the doctor to monitor progress, adjust medications or treatment plans as needed, and address any new concerns.
- **Ask Questions:** Do not hesitate to ask questions about the follow-up care plan. Understanding the recommendations will help you support your loved one's recovery journey.

Working with the Care Team:

- **Open Communication:** Maintain open communication with the doctor, therapist, and any other healthcare professionals involved in your loved one's care.
- **Share Information:** Provide the care team with relevant updates on your loved one's progress at home, including any challenges they might be facing or any improvements they've made.
- **Be an Advocate:** Do not be afraid to voice your concerns or ask questions on behalf of your loved one.

Additional Tips:

- **Keep Medical Records Organized:** Maintain a file or folder to keep all medical records, test results, and medication information organized for easy reference.
- **Refill Medications on Time:** Ensure timely refills of all prescribed medications to avoid any interruptions in treatment.

- **Take Advantage of Support Groups:** Connecting with support groups for stroke survivors and caregivers can provide valuable information, emotional support, and a sense of community.

Remember: Consistent follow-up care is crucial for a successful recovery after a stroke. By managing appointments effectively, understanding the care plan, and working collaboratively with the care team, you can ensure your loved one receives the support they need to heal and regain their independence.

Financial Aid and Insurance Considerations

A stroke can be a life-changing event, not just physically, but financially as well. The cost of medical care, therapy, and potential modifications to your home can add up quickly. This chapter will guide you through understanding insurance coverage, exploring financial aid options, and creating a plan to manage the financial impact of a stroke.

Understanding Insurance Coverage:

Imagine insurance as a safety net that catches some of the financial burden of medical care. Here is what you need to know:

- **Types of Insurance:** There are different types of insurance, like Medicare, Medicaid, or private health insurance. Each has its own coverage details and limitations.
- **Review Your Plan:** Carefully review your insurance plan to understand what's covered related to stroke treatment, therapy, and rehabilitation.
- **Pre-Authorizations:** Some procedures or medications might require pre-authorization from the insurance company before coverage is approved.

Exploring Financial Aid Options:

Financial aid programs can offer assistance with healthcare costs depending on your income and situation. Here are some resources to explore:

- **Government Programs:** Programs like Medicaid or Medicare may offer some financial assistance for stroke-related care.
- **Social Security Disability:** If the stroke has significantly impacted your loved one's ability to work, they might be eligible for Social Security disability benefits.
- **Stroke-Specific Organizations:** Some organizations offer financial assistance programs specifically for stroke survivors.

Managing the Costs:

- **Keep Records:** Maintain clear records of all medical bills and receipts. This will be helpful when dealing with insurance companies or applying for financial aid.
- **Explore Payment Options:** Many hospitals and healthcare providers offer payment plans to help manage the financial burden.
- **Consider Cost-Saving Measures:** Look for ways to reduce costs, like exploring generic medications or seeking support groups for emotional support instead of individual therapy sessions (if applicable based on your loved one's needs and insurance coverage).

Planning for the Future:

- **Long-Term Care Insurance:** Consider talking to a financial advisor about long-term care insurance options to help manage potential future costs related to ongoing care needs.
- **Emergency Fund:** Building an emergency fund can provide a safety net for unexpected medical expenses.
- **Open Communication:** Have open communication with your loved one about finances. Discuss their concerns and work together to create a manageable plan.

Remember: The financial impact of a stroke can be stressful, but there are resources available to help. By understanding insurance coverage, exploring financial aid options, and planning for the future, you can navigate the financial challenges and focus on your loved one's recovery journey. Do not hesitate to seek help from social workers, financial advisors, or stroke organizations for guidance and support.

Adjusting to Life After Stroke

A stroke can be a life-altering event, not just physically but also emotionally. Imagine your brain as the control center for your feelings. A stroke can disrupt this center, leading to a range of emotions like fear, frustration, sadness, or anger. This chapter will guide you on understanding these emotions, coping mechanisms, and finding support for the emotional journey after a stroke.

A Spectrum of Emotions:

It is normal for stroke survivors to experience a wide range of emotions after the event. Here are some common feelings:

- **Fear:** The fear of another stroke, disability, or dependence on others is a common concern.
- **Frustration:** Regaining lost skills or struggling with daily tasks can be frustrating.
- **Sadness:** Loss of independence, changes in appearance, or limitations can lead to sadness or grief.
- **Anger:** Anger at the stroke itself, the limitations it brings, or feelings of helplessness are understandable.

Finding Healthy Coping Mechanisms:

Healthy coping mechanisms can help stroke survivors navigate their emotions. Here are some tips:

- **Talk It Out:** Encourage your loved one to talk about their feelings with a trusted friend, family member, therapist, or support group.
- **Join a Support Group:** Connecting with other stroke survivors can provide emotional support and a sense of community.
- **Relaxation Techniques:** Practices like deep breathing exercises, meditation, or yoga can help manage stress and anxiety.
- **Focus on Achievements:** Celebrate even small victories and milestones on the road to recovery.

The Importance of Patience:

Recovery after a stroke takes time. Be patient with your loved one and yourself. Here are some additional tips:

- **Set Realistic Expectations:** Do not expect immediate improvement. Celebrate progress, no matter how small.
- **Focus on What You Can Control:** Focus on the things you can control, like healthy habits, positive thinking, and a supportive environment.
- **Seek Professional Help:** If emotional struggles become overwhelming, consider seeking professional help from a therapist or counselor specializing in stroke recovery.

Remember: Emotional adjustment after a stroke is a normal part of the healing process. By understanding the common emotions, exploring coping mechanisms, and offering support, you can help your loved one navigate this emotional rollercoaster and build resilience on their journey to recovery.

Discharge Planning and Communication with the Hospital

Imagine you are finally ready to leave the hospital after a stroke. It is exciting to go home, but also a bit scary. There is a lot to think about. This chapter will guide you through discharge planning, a process that helps ensure a smooth transition back home and sets you up for successful recovery.

The Discharge Planning Team:

Think of the discharge planning team as your all-star team for going home. They include:

- **Doctor:** They'll lead the team, explaining your condition, medications, and follow-up care plan.
- **Nurse:** They'll provide instructions on medication management, wound care (if any), and activity restrictions.
- **Social Worker:** They'll connect you with resources like home care services, transportation options, or support groups.
- **Therapist:** They might recommend exercises or adaptive equipment to help you regain independence in daily activities.

Communication is Key:

- **Ask Questions:** Do not hesitate to ask questions - big or small. Understanding your condition and the discharge plan is crucial.
- **Speak Up:** If something is unclear or you have concerns, voice them. The team is there to address your needs.
- **Bring a Support Person:** Consider having a family member or friend present during discharge planning meetings to take notes and ask questions on your behalf.

Preparing for Home:

- **Medications:** Understand your medications, dosages, and side effects. Make sure you have refills arranged before leaving the hospital.
- **Home Modifications:** If your home needs adjustments for safety or accessibility, discuss them with the therapist and make arrangements before going home.

- **Follow-Up Appointments:** Schedule follow-up appointments with your doctor and therapists to monitor your progress.

Additional Tips:

- **Get it in Writing:** Ask for a written copy of your discharge instructions, medication list, and follow-up care plan for future reference.
- **Pack Essentials:** Pack comfortable clothes, toiletries, and any medications you will need at home.
- **Prepare Your Home:** Make sure your home environment is safe and comfortable for recovery. Remove clutter, arrange furniture for easy movement, and ensure good lighting.

Remember: Discharge planning is a collaborative effort. By actively communicating with the hospital team, asking questions, and preparing for home, you can ensure a smooth transition and set yourself up for a successful recovery journey after stroke.

Adapting Transportation Needs After Stroke

Imagine your car is your independence, but after a stroke, getting behind the wheel might not be an immediate option. This chapter will guide you through adapting your transportation needs to ensure you can still get where you need to go safely and conveniently.

Assessing Your Needs:

The first step is to understand your limitations. Here are some things to consider:

- **Physical Ability:** Can you safely operate a vehicle with your current strength, coordination, and vision?
- **Cognitive Functioning:** Can you make sound decisions and react quickly enough while driving?

- **Doctor's Recommendation:** Your doctor will assess your overall health and ability to drive safely.

Exploring Transportation Options:

Once you understand your limitations, you can explore alternative transportation options:

- **Public Transportation:** Buses, trains, or subways can be a convenient and affordable option in some areas.
- **Ridesharing Services:** Apps like Uber or Lyft offer on-demand rides, although costs can add up.
- **Non-Emergency Medical Transportation (NEMT):** Some medical insurance plans may cover transportation to doctor's appointments or therapy sessions.

Regaining Independence Behind the Wheel:

If your goal is to drive again, here are some steps you can take:

- **Occupational Therapy:** An occupational therapist can assess your driving skills and recommend adaptive equipment or training programs to help you regain independence behind the wheel.
- **Vehicle Modifications:** Hand controls, swivel seats, or other modifications might make driving safer and easier.
- **Driver's Re-evaluation:** Your state's Department of Motor Vehicles (DMV) might require a re-evaluation to ensure your fitness to drive.

Planning for the Future:

- **Long-Term Care Options:** Consider future transportation needs as you recover. Explore options like senior transportation services or living in a walkable community.

- **Carpooling or Sharing Rides:** Carpool with friends, family, or neighbors for errands or social outings.
- **Staying Active and Involved:** Maintaining an active lifestyle and social connections can help you stay independent even with limitations in transportation.

Remember: Adapting your transportation needs after a stroke does not mean giving up your independence. By exploring various options, planning for the future, and seeking help from professionals, you can find ways to get around safely and continue living a fulfilling life.

3. PHYSICAL THERAPY AND REHABILITATION

Importance of Physical Therapy After Stroke

Imagine a stroke as a storm that disrupts the smooth flow of messages in your brain. This can affect your movement, coordination, and balance. Physical therapy after a stroke is like sunshine after the storm. It helps your brain relearn how to control your body and regain your independence.

Why is Physical Therapy Important?

Physical therapy is a crucial part of stroke recovery. Here is why:

- **Retraining the Brain:** After a stroke, your brain needs to relearn how to send signals to your muscles. Physical therapists use specific exercises to help your brain create new pathways and regain control over movement.
- **Improving Strength and Coordination:** Stroke can weaken your muscles and affect your coordination. Physical therapy helps strengthen weakened muscles and improve your ability to move smoothly and efficiently.
- **Enhancing Balance:** Balance problems are common after a stroke. Physical therapists design exercises to improve your balance and coordination, making you feel more confident and reducing the risk of falls.
- **Relearning Daily Activities:** Physical therapists can teach you strategies to perform daily tasks safely and independently like dressing, bathing, or getting in and out of bed.

What to Expect in Physical Therapy:

Physical therapy sessions are tailored to your specific needs and abilities. Here is what you might experience:

- **Assessments:** The therapist will assess your strength, movement patterns, balance, and any limitations you might have.
- **Personalized Exercises:** Based on the assessment, the therapist will create a personalized exercise program that gradually increases in difficulty as you progress.
- **Education and Training:** The therapist will educate you on how to perform the exercises safely and effectively at home. They might also train you in using adaptive equipment that can help with daily activities.
- **Motivation and Support:** Physical therapists are your cheerleaders on the road to recovery. They will provide encouragement, celebrate your progress, and help you stay motivated throughout the process.

Benefits of Physical Therapy:

The benefits of physical therapy after stroke go beyond physical improvement. Here is what you might experience:

- **Increased Independence:** Physical therapy empowers you to regain independence in daily activities, boosting your confidence and self-esteem.
- **Reduced Pain:** Stroke can cause muscle stiffness and pain. Physical therapy exercises can help improve flexibility and reduce pain.
- **Improved Quality of Life:** By regaining your strength, mobility, and independence, you can participate more fully in life's activities and improve your overall quality of life.

Remember: Physical therapy is a vital part of stroke recovery. It is never too late to start. With dedication and support from your physical therapist, you can regain control over your body and live a more fulfilling life after stroke.

Exercises for Improving Mobility and Strength

Regaining mobility and strength after a stroke is like teaching your body a new language. It takes practice and patience, but with the right exercises, you can rebuild your strength and move with more confidence. This chapter will guide you through some basic exercises you can do at home to improve mobility and strength after a stroke.

Important Safety Reminders:

- **Listen to Your Body:** Do not push yourself too hard. Start slowly and gradually increase the difficulty of the exercises as you get stronger.
- **Focus on Form:** Proper form is crucial to prevent injury. If an exercise feels uncomfortable or painful, stop and consult your doctor or physical therapist.
- **Warm-Up and Cool-Down:** Always begin with a light warm-up like gentle stretches and end with cool-down exercises to relax your muscles.

Exercises for Improved Mobility:

- **Ankle Circles:** Sit in a chair and slowly rotate your ankles in circles, 10 times in each direction. This improves ankle flexibility.
- **Arm Circles:** Stand with your feet shoulder-width apart and make small circles with your arms, forward and backward 10 times each direction. This improves shoulder mobility.
- **Trunk Twists:** Sit in a chair and gently twist your torso from side to side, reaching as far as comfortably possible. Hold for a few seconds and repeat 10 times on each side. This improves core stability and trunk rotation.

Exercises for Increased Strength:

- **Leg Raises:** Lie on your back with knees bent and feet flat on the floor. Slowly lift one leg straight up, hold for a few seconds, and then lower it back down. Repeat 10 times on each leg. This strengthens your quadriceps.
- **Wall Pushes:** Stand facing a wall with your feet shoulder-width apart. Lean forward slightly and place your hands flat on the wall at shoulder height. Slowly push yourself away from the wall and then return to the starting position. Repeat 10 times. This strengthens your chest, shoulders, and triceps.
- **Heel Lifts:** Stand with your feet shoulder-width apart and hold onto a sturdy chair for balance. Slowly lift your heels off the ground, hold for a few seconds, and then lower them back down. Repeat 10 times. This strengthens your calf muscles.

Progression and Modifications:

As you get stronger, you can gradually increase the difficulty of these exercises. Here are some ways to progress:

- **Increase repetitions:** Once you can comfortably perform 10 repetitions of an exercise, try doing 12 or 15.
- **Add weights:** You can use light weights like water bottles or soup cans to add an extra challenge.
- **Hold for longer:** As your strength improves, hold each exercise position for a longer duration.

Remember: These are just a few examples, and it is crucial to consult with your doctor or physical therapist before starting any exercise program after a stroke. They can create a personalized plan based on your specific needs and limitations.

Additional Tips:

- **Make it Fun:** Find exercises you enjoy and incorporate them into your daily routine.
- **Set Realistic Goals:** Start with small, achievable goals and celebrate your progress along the way.
- **Do not Give Up:** Recovering from a stroke takes time and dedication. Stay motivated and focus on the progress you are making.

By incorporating these exercises into your daily routine, you can improve your mobility, rebuild strength, and rediscover the joy of movement after a stroke.

Spasticity Management

Imagine your muscles are like rubber bands, and after a stroke, some of them might become too tight and stiff. This is called spasticity. It can make movement difficult and uncomfortable. This chapter will explain what spasticity is, how it affects you, and different ways to manage it, helping you regain control and improve your comfort.

What is Spasticity?

Spasticity is a common symptom after stroke. It happens when damage to the part of the brain that controls muscle movement disrupts the communication between the brain and the muscles. This can cause the muscles to become stiff and tight, making it difficult to control your movements.

How Does Spasticity Affect You?

Spasticity can affect you in several ways:

- **Muscle stiffness and tightness:** This can make it difficult to move your arms or legs smoothly.
- **Pain and discomfort:** Tight muscles can be painful and make daily activities challenging.
- **Muscle spasms:** Spasms are sudden involuntary muscle contractions that can be jerky and painful.
- **Limited mobility:** Spasticity can restrict your range of movement, making it difficult to walk, dress, or perform daily tasks.

Managing Spasticity:

The good news is that there are ways to manage spasticity and improve your comfort and mobility. Here are some common approaches:

- **Physical Therapy:** Exercises designed by a physical therapist can help stretch and loosen tight muscles, improve flexibility, and increase your range of motion.
- **Medications:** Certain medications can help relax muscles and reduce spasticity. Your doctor will determine the best medication for you based on your specific needs.
- **Botox injections:** Injecting botulinum toxin (Botox) into specific muscles can temporarily relax them and reduce spasticity.
- **Splints or braces:** These can help support your limbs and prevent muscle contractures (permanent shortening of muscles).
- **Heat therapy:** Applying heat to tight muscles can help relax them and improve flexibility.

Remember: Spasticity management is a collaborative effort. Talk to your doctor or physical therapist about the best approach for you. They can create a personalized plan to address your specific needs and help you regain control and improve your comfort after a stroke.

Additional Tips:

- **Maintain a healthy lifestyle:** Eating a balanced diet, staying hydrated, and getting enough sleep can all contribute to better muscle health and potentially reduce spasticity.
- **Manage stress:** Stress can worsen spasticity. Relaxation techniques like deep breathing or meditation can help manage stress and improve overall well-being.
- **Stay positive:** A positive attitude can go a long way in the recovery process. Focus on the progress you are making and celebrate your achievements.

By understanding spasticity and working with your healthcare team, you can find effective ways to manage it and live a more comfortable and fulfilling life after a stroke.

Balance and Coordination Exercises

After a stroke, regaining your balance and coordination might feel like learning to walk all over again. But do not worry, with a little practice and the right exercises, you can build your confidence and move with more stability. This chapter will guide you through some basic exercises you can do at home to improve your balance and coordination after a stroke.

Why are Balance and Coordination Important?

Balance and coordination are crucial for everyday activities. They allow you to walk safely, climb stairs, reach for objects, and prevent falls.

Important Safety Reminders:

- **Start Slowly and Gradually Progress:** Do not push yourself too hard. Begin with simple exercises and increase difficulty as you gain confidence.

- **Find a Safe Environment:** Practice your exercises in a clear area with plenty of space to move around. Have a sturdy chair or wall nearby for support if needed.
- **Listen to Your Body:** If you feel dizzy or off-balance, stop the exercise and rest. Do not hesitate to ask your doctor or physical therapist for modifications.

Exercises to Improve Balance:

- **Heel-to-Toe Walking:** Walk slowly with your heel of one foot touching the toes of the other foot. Take small steps and focus on maintaining your balance.
- **Single Leg Stands:** Hold onto a sturdy chair or wall for support. Slowly lift one leg off the ground and hold for a few seconds. Repeat on the other side. Gradually increase the hold time as you get stronger.
- **Walking on Different Surfaces:** Once comfortable, try walking on softer surfaces like pillows or a yoga mat to challenge your balance further.

Exercises to Enhance Coordination:

- **Reaching Exercises:** Stand with your feet shoulder-width apart. Slowly reach out with one arm in front of you, then to the side, and then overhead. Repeat with the other arm. Focus on smooth and controlled movements.
- **Ball Transfers:** Sit in a chair and hold a small ball in your hand. Try transferring the ball from one hand to the other without dropping it. This helps with hand-eye coordination.
- **Coin Pick-Up:** Scatter some coins on the floor. Sit in a chair and try picking them up one by one, using only one hand at a time. This improves dexterity and coordination.

Additional Tips:

- **Incorporate Balance into Daily Activities:** Look for opportunities to practice balance throughout the day. For example, try brushing your teeth on one leg or standing on one leg while putting on your socks.
- **Visual Aids:** Use visual markers like lines on the floor or cones to guide your walking and improve balance awareness.
- **Make it Fun:** Choose exercises you enjoy and incorporate them into your daily routine. Play music or watch TV while you exercise to make it more engaging.

Remember: These are just a few examples, and it is crucial to consult with your doctor or physical therapist before starting any exercise program after a stroke. They can create a personalized plan based on your specific needs and limitations.

By practicing these exercises regularly, you can improve your balance, coordination, and confidence in your movements. This will help you regain independence and navigate daily activities with more ease after a stroke.

Assistive Devices for Daily Living

Imagine you are struggling to button your shirt after a stroke. It can be frustrating. But do not worry, there are tools and gadgets called assistive devices that can lend a helping hand and make daily activities easier. This chapter will explore different assistive devices that can improve your independence and quality of life after a stroke.

What are Assistive Devices?

Assistive devices are any tools, equipment, or modifications that help people with disabilities perform daily tasks. They can range from simple and inexpensive items to more complex and technologically advanced tools.

Benefits of Assistive Devices:

- **Increased Independence:** Assistive devices can help you regain independence in daily activities like dressing, bathing, eating, or getting around.
- **Improved Safety:** Certain devices can help prevent falls or injuries, promoting safety in your daily routine.
- **Enhanced Quality of Life:** By making daily tasks easier, assistive devices can improve your confidence and overall quality of life.

Types of Assistive Devices for Daily Living:

- **Reaching Devices:** Long-handled grabbers can help you retrieve objects from high shelves or off the floor.
- **Dressing Aids:** Button extenders, sock aids, or long-handled shoe horns can make dressing easier.
- **Bathroom Safety:** Grab bars, shower chairs, or elevated toilet seats can increase safety and independence in the bathroom.
- **Eating and Drinking Aids:** Weighted utensils, plates with raised edges, or spill-proof cups can make mealtimes less frustrating.
- **Mobility Aids:** Canes, walkers, or wheelchairs can provide support and stability for walking or getting around.

Choosing the Right Assistive Device:

The best assistive device for you depends on your specific needs and limitations. Here are some tips for choosing:

- **Consult Your Therapist:** Talk to your occupational therapist. They can assess your needs and recommend the most appropriate devices for you.

- **Consider Your Needs:** Think about the activities you struggle with the most and choose devices that can help you with those tasks.
- **Try Before You Buy:** If possible, try out different devices before purchasing one to ensure it is comfortable and easy to use.

Additional Tips:

- **Adapt Your Environment:** In addition to assistive devices, consider making changes to your home environment to improve accessibility. For example, install grab bars in the bathroom or remove clutter from walkways.
- **Do not Be Afraid to Ask for Help:** There is no shame in using assistive devices. They are there to help you live a more independent and fulfilling life.
- **Embrace New Technologies:** Explore new and innovative assistive technologies that can further improve your independence.

Remember: Assistive devices are not a sign of weakness; they are tools for empowerment. By using the right devices and adapting your environment, you can overcome challenges and live a more independent life after a stroke.

Regaining Independence in Daily Activities

After a stroke, even basic tasks like getting dressed, showering, or using the restroom can feel overwhelming. But with practice and some helpful techniques, you can regain your independence in these daily activities (ADLs). This chapter will guide you through strategies and tools to make dressing, bathing, and toileting easier and safer after a stroke.

Dressing:

Imagine getting dressed in the morning used to be a breeze, but now it feels like a puzzle. Here are some tips to simplify dressing:

- **Plan Ahead:** Lay out your clothes the night before, choosing loose-fitting garments that are easy to put on and take off. Button-down shirts and pants with elastic waistbands might be easier to manage.
- **Start with the Easier Side:** If you have weakness on one side of your body, dress the stronger side first.
- **Use Assistive Devices:** Button extenders, long-handled shoe horns, or sock aids can make dressing a breeze.
- **Practice Makes Perfect:** The more you practice dressing techniques, the easier and faster it will become.

Bathing:

Taking a shower should be a relaxing experience, not a challenge. Here is how to make it safer and more manageable:

- **Install Grab Bars:** Having grab bars in the shower or bathtub can provide stability and prevent falls.
- **Use a Shower Chair:** A sturdy shower chair allows you to sit comfortably while bathing.
- **Consider a Hand-Held Showerhead:** A hand-held showerhead gives you more control and makes it easier to reach all areas of your body.
- **Non-Slip Mats:** Place non-slip mats in the bathtub or shower to prevent slipping.

Toileting:

Using the restroom should be a private and dignified experience. Here are some ways to make it easier after a stroke:

- **Raised Toilet Seat:** A raised toilet seat can make it easier to sit down and stand up.
- **Grab Bars:** Grab bars near the toilet can provide extra support.
- **Wiping Aids:** Long-handled toilet wipes can be helpful if you have limited mobility.
- **Adaptations for Clothing:** Consider clothing with easy-open closures or adult diapers for managing incontinence if needed.

Remember: Do not be afraid to ask for help. A loved one, caregiver, or occupational therapist can assist you with these tasks and teach you strategies to become more independent.

Additional Tips:

- **Break Down the Tasks:** Think of each activity as a series of smaller steps. Focus on completing one step at a time.
- **Conserve Energy:** Plan your ADLs throughout the day to avoid getting too tired. Take breaks whenever needed.
- **Celebrate Your Progress:** No matter how small, acknowledge your achievements in regaining independence.

By following these tips and practicing regularly, you can overcome challenges and confidently manage your daily activities after a stroke. Remember, regaining independence is a journey, and with patience and determination, you can get there.

Fall Prevention Strategies

A stroke can affect your balance and coordination, making you more prone to falls. But fear not. By implementing fall prevention strategies, you can significantly reduce your risk and live a safer, more independent life. This chapter will guide you through practical tips and helpful tools to keep you on your feet after stroke.

Why is Fall Prevention Important?

Falls can be serious, especially after a stroke. They can lead to injuries like broken bones, head trauma, and a loss of confidence. Fall prevention is crucial for your safety and overall well-being.

Understanding Your Risk Factors:

Knowing your risk factors for falls is the first step towards prevention. Here are some common factors to consider:

- **Balance and Coordination Problems:** Stroke can affect your balance and coordination, making you more likely to lose your footing.
- **Muscle Weakness:** Weak muscles can make it difficult to stand or walk steadily.
- **Vision Impairment:** Blurry vision or difficulty judging distances can increase your fall risk.
- **Medications:** Certain medications can cause dizziness or lightheadedness, leading to falls.

Tips to Reduce Your Fall Risk:

- **Strengthen Your Muscles:** Regular physical therapy exercises can improve your balance, coordination, and muscle strength, making you more stable.
- **Improve Your Home Environment:** Remove clutter from walkways, secure loose rugs, and improve lighting throughout your home.
- **Wear Appropriate Footwear:** Choose well-fitting, closed-toe shoes with good traction to prevent slipping.
- **Use Assistive Devices:** Consider canes, walkers, or grab bars for added support when walking or transferring.
- **See Your Doctor Regularly:** Regular checkups can help identify and manage any medical conditions that could contribute to falls.

- **Talk to Your Pharmacist:** Review your medications with your pharmacist to see if any side effects could increase your fall risk.

Making Daily Activities Safer:

- **Take Your Time:** Do not rush when getting up from a chair or walking. Take your time and focus on maintaining your balance.
- **Ask for Help:** Do not hesitate to ask for help from a loved one or caregiver when needed, especially for tasks that require reaching or climbing.
- **Practice Good Lighting:** Make sure your home is well-lit, especially at night, to avoid tripping over obstacles.

Additional Tips:

- **Maintain a Healthy Lifestyle:** Eat a balanced diet, get enough sleep, and stay hydrated. These habits contribute to overall well-being and can reduce your fall risk.
- **Practice Healthy Habits:** Limit alcohol consumption, which can impair balance and coordination.
- **Be Mindful of the Weather:** Be extra cautious when walking on icy or wet surfaces.

Remember: Fall prevention is a collaborative effort. Talk to your doctor, physical therapist, and occupational therapist. They can assess your individual needs and create a personalized fall prevention plan to keep you safe and independent after stroke. With a proactive approach and a bit of caution, you can significantly reduce your fall risk and live a fulfilling life after stroke.

Pain Management After Stroke

Imagine a constant throb or ache after a stroke. It can be frustrating and make it difficult to participate in therapy or daily activities. This chapter will guide you through understanding pain after stroke, different pain management strategies, and finding relief to improve your quality of life.

Why Does Pain Happen After Stroke?

Pain after a stroke can occur for several reasons:

- **Damaged Tissue:** The stroke itself can damage tissues in the brain or body, leading to pain.
- **Muscle Spasticity:** Tight and stiff muscles, a common symptom after stroke, can cause pain and discomfort.
- **Inflammation:** Stroke can trigger inflammation in the body, contributing to pain.
- **Emotional Distress:** The stress and anxiety following a stroke can sometimes manifest as physical pain.

Types of Pain After Stroke:

- **Neuropathic Pain:** This burning, tingling, or shooting pain results from damage to the nerves.
- **Musculoskeletal Pain:** Muscle stiffness, tightness, or spasms can cause aches and pain.
- **Headaches:** Headaches can occur after a stroke, especially if there was bleeding in the brain.

Managing Pain After Stroke:

The good news is that there are ways to manage pain and improve your comfort after a stroke. Here are some approaches:

- **Medications:** Your doctor might prescribe pain medication, such as over-the-counter pain relievers or stronger medications for neuropathic pain.

- **Physical Therapy:** Exercises designed by a physical therapist can help stretch tight muscles, improve flexibility, and reduce pain associated with spasticity.
- **Heat or Cold Therapy:** Applying heat or cold packs to the affected area can help relieve pain and inflammation.
- **Massage Therapy:** Massage can relax muscles, improve circulation, and reduce pain.
- **Relaxation Techniques:** Practices like meditation, deep breathing, or yoga can help manage stress and anxiety, which can sometimes contribute to perceived pain.

Remember: Communicate with your doctor about your pain. The type, location, and severity of pain all play a role in finding the most effective management strategy.

Additional Tips:

- **Maintain a Healthy Lifestyle:** Eating a balanced diet, getting enough sleep, and staying hydrated can contribute to overall well-being and potentially reduce pain perception.
- **Mind-Body Techniques:** Explore techniques like mindfulness meditation or guided imagery to help manage pain and promote relaxation.
- **Stay Positive:** A positive attitude can go a long way in managing pain and improving your overall well-being.

Living with Pain Does not Have to Be the Norm

By understanding the causes of pain after stroke, communicating openly with your doctor, and exploring different pain management strategies, you can find relief and improve your quality of life. Working with your healthcare team, you can develop a personalized plan to manage pain effectively and live a fulfilling life after stroke.

Speech and Swallowing Therapy

Imagine a stroke affecting the way you talk and swallow. It can be scary and frustrating. But there is good news. Two special therapists, a Speech-Language Pathologist (SLP) and a Swallowing Therapist, can work together like a well-rehearsed dance team to help you regain your voice and swallow safely after a stroke.

Why Work Together?

Stroke can affect your communication and swallowing in different ways. Here is why these therapists are a perfect team:

- **Same Goal, Different Skills:** Both SLPs and Swallowing Therapists want the same thing: to help you communicate clearly and swallow safely after a stroke. But they each have unique skills. SLPs focus on speech and language, while Swallowing Therapists focus on safe swallowing techniques.
- **Complete Picture:** Working together, they get the whole picture. The SLP can identify problems with speaking and understanding words, while the Swallowing Therapist checks if your throat muscles work well for swallowing.
- **Early Intervention:** Catching swallowing problems early is crucial. By working together, they can identify issues and prevent complications like choking on food or drink.

What Does a Speech-Language Pathologist Do?

- **Talk It Out:** The SLP will assess your speech and language skills. They might ask you to name pictures, repeat sentences, or answer questions.
- **Treatment Time:** Based on the assessment, the SLP creates a personalized plan to address your specific needs. This might

involve exercises to improve how you form sounds, strengthen your voice, or help you find new ways to communicate.

What Does a Swallowing Therapist Do?

- **Swallow Check:** The Swallowing Therapist will assess your swallowing ability. This might involve checking your mouth and throat or using a special x-ray test to see how you swallow.
- **Safe Swallowing:** Based on the assessment, they will develop a safe swallowing plan. This might involve exercises to strengthen your swallowing muscles, changing the texture of your food, or learning special techniques to swallow safely.
- **Diet Talk:** The Swallowing Therapist might recommend temporary or permanent changes to your diet to ensure safe swallowing.

Benefits of Teamwork:

- **Talk and Swallow with Confidence:** By addressing both speech and swallowing issues, you can regain your ability to communicate clearly and enjoy meals safely.
- **Fewer Worries:** Early identification and treatment of swallowing problems can prevent you from choking on food or drink.
- **Better Days Ahead:** Effective communication and safe swallowing contribute significantly to a happier and healthier life after a stroke.

Remember: Communication is key. Be open with your SLP and Swallowing Therapist about any challenges you are facing. They work as a team to create a recovery plan just for you.

Extra Tips:

- **Family Support:** Involve your family in understanding your communication and swallowing needs. Their support can make a big difference.
- **Patience is Key:** Recovery takes time and effort. Be patient with yourself and celebrate every step forward.
- **Positive Thinking:** A positive attitude can be powerful. Focus on the improvements you are making.

By working together as a team, SLPs and Swallowing Therapists can play a vital role in helping you regain your voice, swallow safely, and improve your overall quality of life after a stroke.

Physical Therapy Techniques for Stroke Recovery

After a stroke, your body might feel stiff, weak, or uncoordinated. But do not worry, physical therapy can help. This chapter will explore different physical therapy techniques used to address specific impairments caused by stroke, such as hemiplegia and ataxia.

Physical Therapy: Your Path to Recovery

Physical therapists are experts in movement and rehabilitation. After a stroke, they will assess your individual needs and create a personalized therapy plan to help you regain strength, flexibility, coordination, and balance. Here is how physical therapy can target specific stroke impairments:

Hemiplegia: This is a condition where one side of your body is paralyzed or weak after a stroke. Here are some techniques used to address hemiplegia:

- **Strengthening Exercises:** Exercises designed to target the weakened muscles on the affected side. This can help improve muscle strength and function.
- **Range-of-Motion Exercises:** Gentle stretches to improve flexibility and prevent joint stiffness in the affected limbs.
- **Balance and Coordination Training:** Exercises that challenge your balance and coordination, helping you move both sides of your body together more effectively.
- **Neuromotor Retraining:** Techniques that stimulate the brain to relearn movement patterns on the affected side. This can involve repetitive practice of specific tasks or using special equipment.

Ataxia: This condition causes problems with balance, coordination, and speech after a stroke. Here are some techniques used to address ataxia:

- **Gait Training:** Exercises to improve your walking pattern, such as walking on different surfaces or practicing with assistive devices like canes or walkers.
- **Balance Exercises:** Activities that challenge your sense of balance, helping you regain stability and prevent falls.
- **Proprioceptive Training:** Exercises that help you become more aware of your body position in space. This can improve your coordination and movement control.
- **Sensory Integration Techniques:** Activities that stimulate different senses, such as visual or auditory cues, to help improve your brain's ability to process information and coordinate movement.

Remember: These are just some examples, and the specific techniques used will vary depending on your individual needs and the severity of your stroke.

Additional Considerations:

- **Spasticity Management:** Physical therapists can also help manage muscle stiffness (spasticity) that can occur after a stroke. This might involve stretching exercises, splinting, or medication.
- **Functional Training:** Physical therapy focuses not just on isolated movements, but also on helping you regain the ability to perform daily activities like dressing, bathing, and self-care.
- **Pain Management:** If you are experiencing pain after a stroke, your physical therapist can incorporate pain management techniques into your therapy plan.

The Road to Recovery

Physical therapy is a crucial part of stroke rehabilitation. It can help you regain strength, coordination, and independence after a stroke. Be patient with yourself, celebrate your progress, and work closely with your physical therapist to achieve your recovery goals.

Here are some additional tips:

- **Practice at Home:** Regular practice of exercises prescribed by your therapist is essential for optimal recovery.
- **Communication is Key:** Open communication with your therapist about any challenges or limitations you face will help them tailor your therapy plan accordingly.
- **Maintain a Healthy Lifestyle:** Eating a balanced diet, getting enough sleep, and staying active can all contribute to a faster and more successful recovery.

By working with your physical therapist and incorporating these strategies, you can overcome challenges and regain control over your movements after a stroke.

Pain Management Techniques

Imagine a constant ache or throb after a stroke. It can be frustrating and make it difficult to participate in therapy or daily activities. But there is good news. Physical therapists have a toolbox full of techniques called "physical therapy modalities" that can help manage pain and improve your comfort after a stroke. This chapter will explore these techniques and how they can help you find relief.

Why Does Pain Happen After Stroke?

There are several reasons why you might experience pain after a stroke:

- **Damaged Tissue:** The stroke itself can damage tissues in the brain or body, leading to pain.
- **Muscle Spasticity:** Tight and stiff muscles, a common symptom after stroke, can cause pain and discomfort.
- **Inflammation:** Stroke can trigger inflammation in the body, contributing to pain.
- **Phantom Limb Pain:** If you have lost a limb due to stroke, you might experience a strange sensation of pain in the missing limb.

Physical Therapy Modalities for Pain Relief:

Physical therapists utilize various modalities to target different types of pain after stroke. Here are some common techniques:

- **Heat Therapy:** Applying warm packs or using moist heat therapy can help relax muscles, improve blood flow, and reduce pain and stiffness.
- **Cold Therapy:** Ice packs or cold therapy can be helpful for acute pain and inflammation. It can also numb the area temporarily, providing pain relief.

- **Electrical Stimulation:** Low-dose electrical currents can help relieve pain by stimulating nerve fibers and blocking pain signals to the brain.
- **Ultrasound Therapy:** Sound waves penetrate deep into tissues, promoting healing, reducing inflammation, and alleviating pain.
- **Massage Therapy:** Massage can relax tight muscles, improve circulation, and reduce pain and discomfort.

Remember: Not all modalities are suitable for everyone. Your physical therapist will assess your specific situation and recommend the most appropriate techniques for your pain relief.

Additional Techniques:

- **Therapeutic Exercises:** Exercises designed to improve flexibility, strengthen muscles, and improve range of motion can all contribute to pain reduction.
- **Posture and Body Mechanics Training:** Learning proper posture and body mechanics can help reduce stress on your joints and muscles, preventing pain.
- **Relaxation Techniques:** Techniques like deep breathing or meditation can help manage stress and anxiety, which can sometimes worsen pain perception.

Working Together for Pain Relief:

Physical therapy modalities are often used alongside other pain management strategies, such as medication or lifestyle changes. It is important to communicate openly with your doctor and physical therapist about your pain. They can work together to create a personalized plan to manage your pain effectively.

Here are some additional tips:

- **Be Patient:** Pain management after stroke takes time and effort. Be patient with yourself and celebrate even small improvements.
- **Listen to Your Body:** Pay attention to your body's signals. If a particular modality seems to worsen your pain, let your therapist know.
- **Maintain a Healthy Lifestyle:** Eating a balanced diet, getting enough sleep, and staying active can all contribute to a faster and more effective pain management plan.

By working with your physical therapist and trying different modalities, you can find relief from pain and improve your overall well-being after stroke. Remember, you do not have to live with constant pain. There are ways to manage it and improve your quality of life.

Aquatic Therapy for Stroke Rehabilitation

Imagine a warm pool where your movements feel lighter and your muscles feel less stiff. That's the magic of aquatic therapy. This chapter will explore how exercising in water can be a beneficial addition to your stroke rehabilitation journey.

Why Aquatic Therapy?

Stroke can affect your strength, mobility, and balance. Aquatic therapy offers a unique environment for rehabilitation with several benefits:

- **Buoyancy:** Water supports your body weight, reducing stress on your joints and muscles. This allows you to move more freely and practice exercises that might be difficult on land.
- **Warmth:** The warm water can help relax tight muscles, improve blood flow, and reduce pain, making exercise more comfortable.
- **Resistance:** The water provides gentle resistance as you move, helping strengthen your muscles and improve coordination.

- **Confidence Booster:** The buoyancy and support of water can boost your confidence and motivation to exercise, leading to better engagement in therapy.

How Does Aquatic Therapy Work?

Aquatic therapy sessions are conducted in a warm pool by a specially trained physical therapist. The therapist will create a personalized exercise program based on your needs and goals. These exercises can include:

- **Walking:** Walking in shallow water challenges your balance and builds leg strength.
- **Range-of-Motion Exercises:** Gentle stretches in the water improve flexibility and reduce muscle stiffness.
- **Strengthening Exercises:** Exercises with water resistance bands or other equipment can help rebuild muscle strength.
- **Balance and Coordination Activities:** Activities that challenge your balance and coordination can be practiced more safely in water.

Benefits of Aquatic Therapy for Stroke Rehabilitation:

- **Improved Mobility:** The combination of buoyancy and resistance helps you move more easily and regain control over your movements.
- **Increased Strength:** Aquatic exercises can help strengthen weakened muscles, improving your overall functional ability.
- **Enhanced Balance:** Exercises in water challenge your balance system, improving stability and reducing fall risk.
- **Reduced Pain:** The warmth and support of water can help manage pain, making therapy more comfortable and enjoyable.

Aquatic Therapy Might Be Right for You If:

- You have difficulty moving on land due to pain or weakness.
- You are afraid of falling during land-based therapy.
- You enjoy exercising in water and find it motivating.

Remember: Aquatic therapy is not a replacement for traditional land-based physical therapy. It is a complementary therapy that can be used alongside other rehabilitation techniques.

Here are some additional tips:

- **Talk to Your Doctor:** Discuss whether aquatic therapy is a suitable addition to your recovery plan.
- **Find a Qualified Therapist:** Look for a therapist certified in aquatic therapy for neurological conditions.
- **Start Slowly and Progress Gradually:** Just like any other form of exercise, start with gentle exercises and gradually increase intensity as you get stronger.

Embrace the Waves of Recovery:

Aquatic therapy can be a fun and effective way to improve your recovery after stroke. By incorporating water exercises into your rehabilitation plan, you can experience increased mobility, improved strength, and a more positive outlook on your journey. So, dive in and experience the benefits of aquatic therapy.

Robotics and Technology-Assisted Rehabilitation

Imagine a future where robots and high-tech gadgets assist you in your stroke rehabilitation journey. Well, that future is already here. This chapter will explore how robotics and technology are playing an increasingly important role in helping people regain strength, mobility, and independence after a stroke.

The Rise of Robotic Therapy:

Stroke can impact movement, coordination, and balance. Robotic therapy offers innovative tools to enhance traditional rehabilitation techniques:

- **Robotic Arms and Exoskeletons:** These robotic devices can provide support and guidance as you move your limbs, helping retrain muscles and improve movement patterns.
- **Virtual Reality (VR) Therapy:** VR creates immersive environments where you can practice tasks like walking through a virtual supermarket or reaching for objects. This can improve motor skills and coordination in a fun and engaging way.
- **Video Games for Therapy:** Interactive video games that challenge your balance, coordination, and cognitive skills can be used as therapeutic tools to improve these functions.
- **Smart Wearables:** Wearable devices like armbands or sensors can track your movements and provide feedback, helping you monitor your progress and optimize your therapy exercises.

Benefits of Technology-Assisted Rehabilitation:

- **Intensified Therapy:** Robots and technology can provide repetitive and intensive therapy sessions, potentially leading to faster improvements.
- **Task-Specific Training:** Technology can simulate real-life activities, allowing you to practice skills you need for daily living.
- **Motivation and Engagement:** Interactive games and virtual environments can make therapy more fun and engaging, encouraging you to participate actively.
- **Biofeedback and Monitoring:** Technology can provide real-time feedback on your performance, allowing you to track progress and adjust your exercises for better results.

Important Considerations:

- **Technology is a Tool:** Robots and technology are not replacements for skilled therapists. They are tools used alongside traditional therapy to enhance your recovery.
- **Not for Everyone:** Technology-assisted therapy might not be suitable for everyone. Your doctor or therapist will assess your needs and determine if it is a good fit for you.
- **Cost and Accessibility:** Technology-based therapy can be expensive and may not be readily available in all healthcare settings.

The Future of Rehabilitation Technology:

The field of rehabilitation robotics and technology is constantly evolving. As technology becomes more affordable and accessible, we can expect even more innovative tools to be developed, offering personalized and effective rehabilitation experiences for stroke survivors.

Here are some additional tips:

- **Talk to Your Therapist:** Discuss whether technology-assisted therapy could benefit your recovery plan.
- **Be Open to Trying New Things:** Embrace the potential of technology to enhance your rehabilitation journey.
- **Focus on Progress:** Celebrate your improvements, big or small, as you work towards your recovery goals.

By incorporating robotics and technology alongside traditional therapy, you can unlock new possibilities for your stroke rehabilitation. With dedication and the right tools, you can regain strength, improve your mobility, and achieve a greater degree of independence after stroke.

4. SPEECH AND LANGUAGE THERAPY

Imagine a stroke affecting the way you think, speak, understand, or even write. It can be scary and frustrating. But the good news is, with practice and support, you can overcome these communication challenges and regain your voice. This chapter will explore the different communication difficulties you might face after a stroke, and strategies to help you communicate effectively.

Effect of Stroke on Communication

A stroke can damage different parts of the brain that control communication. Here are some common challenges you might encounter:

- **Aphasia:** This is a difficulty understanding or using spoken language. You might struggle to find the right words, understand what others are saying, or both.
- **Dysarthria:** This affects the muscles used for speaking. You might slur your words, speak too softly, or have difficulty controlling your voice.
- **Apraxia of Speech:** This makes it hard to coordinate the movements needed for speech. You might know what you want to say, but struggle to form the sounds correctly.
- **Cognitive-Communication Problems:** Stroke can affect your memory, attention, and thinking skills, making it difficult to follow conversations or express yourself clearly.

Do not Give Up. Strategies for Communication After Stroke:

There are many ways to overcome these communication challenges and improve your ability to connect with others:

- **Speech Therapy:** A speech-language pathologist (SLP) can assess your specific communication difficulties and develop a personalized therapy plan to help you relearn speech patterns, improve comprehension, and find alternative communication methods.
- **Practice Makes Progress:** Regularly practicing communication exercises recommended by your SLP can help strengthen your speech skills and improve your confidence.
- **Alternative Communication Methods:** If speaking is difficult, explore tools like picture boards, writing tablets, or communication apps that can help you express yourself.
- **Patience is Key:** Recovery takes time and effort. Be patient with yourself and celebrate small improvements.
- **Communication Strategies:** Your family and friends can help by using clear and simple language, giving you time to respond, and avoiding interrupting you.

Tips for Supporting Someone with Communication Challenges After Stroke:

- **Be Patient and Respectful:** Give them time to process information and respond.
- **Focus on Nonverbal Cues:** Pay attention to facial expressions and gestures to understand their emotions.
- **Use Simple Language:** Speak slowly and clearly, and avoid using complex sentences.
- **Encourage Participation:** Involve them in conversations and offer choices whenever possible.
- **Be Positive and Supportive:** Offer encouragement and celebrate their communication victories.

Remember: Communication is a two-way street. By working together, using the right strategies, and having a positive attitude, you can overcome communication challenges after stroke and continue to connect meaningfully with the world around you.

Additional Tips:

- **Join a Support Group:** Connecting with others who understand your challenges can be very helpful.
- **Stay Connected:** Maintain relationships with family and friends who can support you through your recovery.
- **Maintain a Healthy Lifestyle:** Eating a balanced diet, getting enough sleep, and managing stress can all contribute to improved communication skills.

By following these tips and working with your healthcare team, you can regain your voice and overcome communication challenges after stroke. There is hope for reconnecting with the world and expressing yourself clearly again.

Strategies for Improving Speech and Language

Imagine a stroke affecting your ability to speak clearly or understand what others are saying. It can be frustrating and isolating. But the good news is, with dedication and the right tools, you can regain your communication skills. This chapter explores different strategies to improve your speech and language after a stroke.

Why Does Stroke Affect Communication?

A stroke can damage areas of the brain responsible for language processing. This can lead to difficulties like:

- **Aphasia:** Trouble understanding or using spoken language. You might struggle to find words, follow conversations, or both.
- **Dysarthria:** Weakness or lack of coordination in the muscles used for speaking. This can cause slurred speech, difficulty controlling your voice volume, or problems pronouncing words.

- **Apraxia of Speech:** Inability to coordinate the movements needed for speech, even though you know what you want to say.

Taking Back Your Voice: Strategies for Improvement

There are many effective strategies to help you regain your communication skills after a stroke:

- **Speech Therapy:** A speech-language pathologist (SLP) is your communication champion. They will assess your specific challenges and create a personalized therapy plan. This might involve:
    o Exercises to improve articulation and pronunciation.
    o Activities to enhance your vocabulary and sentence structure.
    o Practice sessions to improve your comprehension of spoken language.
- **Practice Makes Progress:** Regularly practicing the exercises recommended by your SLP is crucial. This might include daily drills, reading aloud, or conversation practice with a therapist or loved ones.
- **Technology Can Help:** There are speech recognition apps, communication software, and other assistive technologies that can aid communication when speaking is difficult.
- **Alternative Communication Methods:** If speaking remains challenging, explore tools like picture boards, writing tablets, or communication apps to express yourself clearly.

Remember: Recovery takes time and effort. Be patient with yourself and celebrate even small improvements. Here are some additional tips:

- **Focus on Nonverbal Communication:** Use gestures, facial expressions, and body language to support your speech.

- **Communication Strategies for Your Partner:** Ask your family and friends to speak slowly and clearly, and to give you time to process information.
- **Join a Support Group:** Connecting with others who understand your challenges can be very encouraging and offer valuable insights.
- **Maintain a Healthy Lifestyle:** A balanced diet, good sleep, and managing stress can all contribute to improved communication skills.

The Road to Recovery

By working with your healthcare team, practicing speech therapy exercises, and using the right strategies, you can overcome communication challenges after a stroke. Remember, regaining your voice is a journey, not a destination. With dedication and a positive attitude, you can improve your speech and language skills, and reconnect with the world around you.

Augmentative and Alternative Communication

Imagine a stroke affecting the way you speak. You might struggle to find the right words or express yourself clearly. This can be frustrating, but there is hope. Augmentative and Alternative Communication (AAC) tools can help you find your voice in new ways and keep you connected with the world.

What is AAC?

AAC refers to any method of communication that supplements or replaces spoken language. It is a toolbox filled with strategies and tools to help people of all ages express themselves when speaking is difficult due to a stroke or other conditions.

Who Can Benefit from AAC?

People with aphasia, dysarthria, or other communication challenges after stroke can benefit from AAC. It can also be helpful for individuals with other conditions that affect speech.

Types of AAC Systems:

There are many different AAC systems available, ranging from low-tech to high-tech. Here are some common types:

- **Low-Tech AAC:** This includes picture boards, communication books, and letter boards. You can point to pictures or letters to form words and sentences.
- **Mid-Tech AAC:** These are electronic devices with pre-recorded messages or symbols that you can choose to express yourself.
- **High-Tech AAC:** These are sophisticated devices with speech synthesis capabilities. You can type words or sentences, and the device will voice them for you.

Choosing the Right AAC System:

The best AAC system for you will depend on your individual needs and preferences. Factors to consider include the severity of your communication challenge, your dexterity, and your comfort level with technology. Your speech-language pathologist (SLP) can help you assess your needs and recommend the most suitable system.

Benefits of Using AAC:

- **Improved Communication:** AAC allows you to express yourself clearly and effectively, even if speaking is difficult.
- **Increased Independence:** With AAC, you can communicate your needs and wants, leading to a greater sense of independence.

- **Enhanced Social Interaction:** AAC helps you participate in conversations and connect with others more effectively.
- **Boosted Confidence:** Being able to communicate your thoughts and feelings can improve your self-esteem and confidence.

Remember: Learning to use AAC takes time and practice. Be patient with yourself and celebrate your progress as you become more comfortable with the system.

Here are some additional tips:

- **Involve Your Family and Friends:** Encourage your loved ones to learn about AAC and how to communicate effectively with you using the system.
- **Practice Regularly:** The more you practice using your AAC system, the more comfortable and confident you will become.
- **Stay Positive:** Focus on the possibilities that AAC opens up for your communication and social interaction.

Finding Your Voice Again

AAC is a powerful tool that can help you overcome communication challenges after stroke. By embracing AAC and exploring different systems, you can find your voice in new ways and continue to express yourself, connect with others, and live a fulfilling life.

Cognitive Rehabilitation: Memory, Attention, and Problem-Solving

Imagine a stroke affecting your ability to remember things, focus on tasks, or solve problems. It can be frustrating and make daily life challenging. But there is good news. Cognitive rehabilitation, also called brain training, can help you regain these skills after a stroke.

The Power of Cognitive Rehabilitation

A stroke can damage parts of the brain responsible for thinking, learning, and memory. Cognitive rehabilitation helps retrain these brain areas and improve your cognitive skills like:

- **Memory:** Remembering names, appointments, or where you placed things.
- **Attention:** Focusing on one task at a time and avoiding distractions.
- **Problem-solving:** Figuring out solutions to challenges you encounter in daily life.
- **Organization:** Planning your day, managing your belongings, and following routines.

How Does Cognitive Rehabilitation Work?

Cognitive rehabilitation is not about memorizing facts. It involves targeted exercises and strategies to retrain your brain:

- **Memory Games:** Activities like remembering sequences, matching pictures, or practicing memory strategies can help strengthen memory pathways.
- **Attention Training:** Computerized exercises or games can help improve your ability to focus and filter out distractions.
- **Problem-Solving Exercises:** Practicing real-life scenarios, such as planning a meal or balancing a budget, can enhance your problem-solving skills.
- **Organization Techniques:** Learning strategies like using calendars, planners, or labeling items can improve your organizational skills.

Benefits of Cognitive Rehabilitation After Stroke:

- **Improved Cognitive Skills:** Regular brain training can help regain your memory, attention, and problem-solving abilities.
- **Enhanced Independence:** With improved cognitive skills, you can manage daily tasks more efficiently and regain your independence.
- **Increased Confidence:** Being able to think clearly and solve problems can boost your confidence and well-being.
- **Better Quality of Life:** Cognitive rehabilitation can significantly improve your overall quality of life after stroke.

Remember: Cognitive rehabilitation takes time and dedication. Be patient with yourself and celebrate small improvements. Here are some additional tips:

- **Work with a Therapist:** A trained therapist can assess your specific needs and create a personalized rehabilitation plan.
- **Practice Makes Progress:** Regularly practicing the exercises recommended by your therapist is crucial for improvement.
- **Incorporate Strategies in Daily Life:** Try to integrate the memory, attention, and problem-solving skills you learn into your daily routines.
- **Maintain a Healthy Lifestyle:** Eating a balanced diet, getting enough sleep, and managing stress can all contribute to improved cognitive function.

Unlocking Your Brain's Potential

Cognitive rehabilitation is a valuable tool for regaining cognitive skills after a stroke. By working with a therapist, practicing exercises diligently, and incorporating helpful strategies into your daily life, you can unlock your brain's potential and improve your memory, attention, and problem-solving abilities. This can lead to greater independence, increased confidence, and a better quality of life after stroke. Remember, your brain is capable of remarkable recovery, and cognitive rehabilitation can help you get there.

Strategies for Communication After Aphasia

Imagine a stroke affecting your ability to understand or use spoken language. It can be scary and isolating. But the good news is, with dedication and the right tools, you can overcome these communication challenges and regain your voice. This chapter explores Aphasia, a common communication difficulty after stroke, and offers strategies to help you connect with the world around you.

Understanding Aphasia

Aphasia is a language disorder caused by stroke damage to the brain regions responsible for processing language. It can affect your ability to:

- **Speak:** Finding the right words, forming sentences, or slurring your speech.
- **Understand:** Difficulty following conversations, misunderstanding what others are saying, or getting confused by complex words.
- **Read:** Struggling to read or understand written words.
- **Write:** Difficulty writing words or sentences correctly.

The Severity Can Vary:

The severity of aphasia can vary depending on the location and extent of the stroke damage. Some people might experience mild difficulties, while others might have a more significant impact on their communication skills.

Do not Give Up. Strategies for Communication

There are many ways to overcome communication challenges after Aphasia and improve your ability to connect with others:

- **Speech Therapy:** A speech-language pathologist (SLP) is your communication champion. They will assess your specific challenges and develop a personalized therapy plan. This might involve:
  - Exercises to improve your ability to find words.
  - Practice sessions to improve your comprehension of spoken language.
  - Strategies to help you express yourself using gestures, facial expressions, or alternative communication methods.
- **Practice Makes Progress:** Regularly practicing the exercises recommended by your SLP is crucial. This might include daily drills, picture communication tools, or conversation practice with a therapist or loved ones.
- **Alternative Communication Methods:** If speaking remains challenging, explore tools like picture boards, communication apps with symbols, or even writing tablets to express yourself clearly.
- **Patience is Key:** Recovery takes time and effort. Be patient with yourself and celebrate even small improvements in your communication skills.

Tips for Supporting Someone with Aphasia:

- **Be Patient and Respectful:** Give them time to process information and respond. Do not finish their sentences or talk too fast.
- **Focus on Nonverbal Cues:** Pay attention to facial expressions and gestures to understand their emotions and intentions.
- **Use Simple Language:** Speak slowly and clearly, and avoid using complex sentences or idioms.

- **Encourage Participation:** Involve them in conversations and offer choices whenever possible.
- **Communication Strategies:** Ask "yes" or "no" questions, use visuals like pictures or objects, and allow them to use alternative communication methods.

Remember: Communication is a two-way street. By working together, using the right strategies, and having a positive attitude, you can overcome communication challenges after Aphasia. There is hope for reconnecting with the world and expressing yourself clearly again.

Additional Tips:

- **Join a Support Group:** Connecting with others who understand your challenges can be very encouraging and offer valuable insights.
- **Maintain a Healthy Lifestyle:** Eating a balanced diet, getting enough sleep, and managing stress can all contribute to improved communication skills.

By following these tips and working with your healthcare team, you can regain your voice and overcome communication challenges after Aphasia. There is light at the end of the tunnel. With dedication and a positive attitude, you can improve your communication skills and live a fulfilling life.

Assistive Technologies for Communication

Imagine a stroke affecting your ability to speak clearly or understand what others are saying. It can be frustrating, but there is hope. Assistive technologies (AT) are like helpful gadgets that can bridge the communication gap after a stroke. This chapter will explore different AT tools to empower you to express yourself and connect with the world.

What are Assistive Technologies for Communication?

AT tools are devices or software designed to help people with communication difficulties. They can be low-tech, like picture boards, or high-tech, like voice synthesizers. Here are some common types:

- **Low-Tech AT:** These are simple and easy-to-use tools that do not require electricity. Examples include:
    - **Picture boards:** Boards with symbols or images that you can point to represent words or ideas.
    - **Communication books:** Books with pre-printed phrases or sentences you can use for common situations.
    - **Letter boards:** Boards with letters that you can point to spell words.
- **Mid-Tech AT:** These electronic devices offer more options and flexibility than low-tech tools. Examples include:
    - **Dedicated communication devices:** These handheld devices have pre-recorded messages or symbols you can choose to express yourself.
    - **Speech-generating software:** Software that allows you to type words or phrases, and the device speaks them for you.
- **High-Tech AT:** These sophisticated devices offer advanced features like voice recognition and text-to-speech capabilities. Examples include:
    - **Tablets with communication apps:** Apps with customizable features like symbol sets, voice output, and text prediction.
    - **Eye-tracking systems:** For people with limited mobility, these systems allow you to control communication software with your eye movements.

Choosing the Right AT for You:

The best AT for you depend on your specific needs and preferences. Factors to consider include the severity of your communication challenge, your dexterity level, and your comfort level with technology. Your speech-language pathologist (SLP) can assess your needs and recommend the most suitable AT options.

Benefits of Using Assistive Technologies:

- **Improved Communication:** AT allows you to express yourself clearly and effectively, even if speaking is difficult.
- **Increased Independence:** With AT, you can communicate your needs and wants, leading to a greater sense of independence.
- **Enhanced Social Interaction:** AT helps you participate in conversations and connect with others more effectively.
- **Boosted Confidence:** Being able to communicate your thoughts and feelings can improve your self-esteem and confidence.

Remember: Learning to use AT takes time and practice. Be patient with yourself and celebrate your progress as you become more comfortable with the technology. Here are some additional tips:

- **Involve Your Family and Friends:** Encourage your loved ones to learn about AT and how to communicate effectively with you using these tools.
- **Practice Regularly:** The more you practice using your AT, the more comfortable and confident you will become.
- **Explore Different Options:** There are many different AT tools available. Do not be afraid to experiment and find what works best for you.

Finding Your Voice Again

Assistive technologies are powerful tools that can help you overcome communication challenges after a stroke. By embracing AT, exploring different options, and working with your therapist, you can find your voice again and continue to express yourself, connect with others, and live a fulfilling life. Remember, technology is here to help you regain your communication power.

Music Therapy for Speech and Language Improvement

Imagine a world where music becomes a bridge to healing your speech and language after a stroke. That's the magic of music therapy. This chapter explores how music can be a powerful tool to improve your communication skills and rediscover your voice.

Why Music Therapy?

Stroke can damage the brain areas responsible for speech and language. Music therapy offers a unique approach to rehabilitation with several benefits:

- **The Brain on Music:** Music activates many areas of the brain, including those involved in speech and language processing. This stimulation can help retrain these areas and promote recovery.
- **Motivation and Engagement:** Music can be fun and engaging, making therapy sessions more enjoyable and increasing your motivation to participate.
- **Melodic Pathways:** Singing songs with specific rhythms and melodies can help improve articulation, fluency, and overall speech production.
- **Memory and Attention Boost:** Music can enhance memory and focus, which are crucial skills for effective communication.

How Does Music Therapy Work?

Music therapy sessions are conducted by a certified music therapist who creates a personalized program based on your needs. Here are some examples of how music can be used:

- **Singing:** Singing exercises can target specific sounds, improve pronunciation, and enhance your breath control for clearer speech.
- **Rhythmic Activities:** Clapping, tapping, or drumming along to music can improve your coordination and sequencing skills, which are important for speech production.
- **Songwriting:** Creating your own songs can be a fun way to practice using words and expressing yourself creatively.
- **Listening and Responding:** Listening attentively to music with varying tempos and rhythms can help improve your auditory processing skills, which are essential for understanding language.

Benefits of Music Therapy for Speech and Language:

- **Improved Speech Production:** Music therapy can help you speak more clearly, with better articulation and fluency.
- **Enhanced Language Comprehension:** Exercises can improve your ability to understand spoken language.
- **Boosted Memory and Attention:** Music therapy can enhance your cognitive skills, which are vital for communication.
- **Increased Confidence:** Experiencing progress in your communication skills can boost your confidence and motivation to continue therapy.

Music Therapy Might Be Right for You If:

- You have difficulty speaking clearly or understanding language after a stroke.

- You struggle to find motivation for traditional speech therapy sessions.
- You enjoy music and find it engaging.

Remember: Music therapy is not a replacement for traditional speech therapy. It is a complementary therapy that can be used alongside other techniques for a more holistic approach to recovery.

Here are some additional tips:

- **Talk to Your Doctor:** Discuss whether music therapy could be a beneficial addition to your rehabilitation plan.
- **Find a Qualified Therapist:** Look for a music therapist certified in working with stroke survivors.
- **Embrace the Journey:** Approach music therapy with an open mind and enjoy the process of rediscovering your voice through music.

The Power of Song

Music therapy can be a powerful tool for improving your communication skills after a stroke. By incorporating music into your therapy plan, you can experience a more enjoyable and engaging recovery journey. So, hum along, tap your toes, and rediscover the rhythm of communication through the magic of music.

5. NUTRITIONAL NEEDS AFTER STROKE

Imagine a stroke affecting your body and leaving you feeling weak. What you eat can play a crucial role in your recovery journey. This chapter explores the importance of proper nutrition after a stroke and how the right foods can help you heal and regain your strength.

Importance of Nutrition After Stroke

Stroke damages parts of the brain, impacting your body's functions, including how you use energy. Proper nutrition ensures your body gets the essential nutrients it needs to:

- **Heal and Repair Tissues:** Stroke damages your brain tissue. Getting enough protein and vitamins helps your body rebuild and repair these damaged areas.
- **Maintain Muscle Strength:** Stroke can lead to muscle weakness. Eating protein-rich foods helps maintain muscle mass and improve your ability to move.
- **Manage Blood Pressure and Cholesterol:** High blood pressure and cholesterol are risk factors for stroke. A healthy diet helps manage these levels and reduce the risk of future strokes.
- **Boost Energy Levels:** Feeling tired after a stroke is common. Eating a balanced diet with complex carbohydrates provides sustained energy throughout the day.

What to Eat After Stroke

Focus on a balanced diet that includes these essential food groups:

- **Fruits and Vegetables:** These are packed with vitamins, minerals, and antioxidants that support healing and overall health.

- **Whole Grains:** Whole-wheat bread, brown rice, and quinoa provide sustained energy and dietary fiber, which is good for digestion.
- **Lean Protein:** Fish, chicken, beans, and lentils provide the building blocks for muscle repair and strength.
- **Healthy Fats:** Omega-3 fatty acids found in fatty fish and nuts promote brain health and may aid recovery.
- **Low-Fat Dairy:** Dairy products provide calcium for bone health and vitamin D, which is essential for overall well-being.

What to Limit After Stroke

Some foods can hinder your recovery and should be limited:

- **Added Sugars and Sweets:** These provide quick energy but can lead to blood sugar spikes and crashes, leaving you feeling tired.
- **Saturated and Trans Fats:** Found in fried foods, processed meats, and pastries, these fats can increase unhealthy cholesterol levels.
- **Added Salt:** Too much salt can raise blood pressure, which is a risk factor for stroke.

Remember: Eating a balanced diet is key, but specific needs may vary based on your condition.

Here are some additional tips:

- **Talk to a Registered Dietitian:** A dietitian can create a personalized meal plan based on your specific needs and preferences.
- **Stay Hydrated:** Drinking plenty of water is crucial for overall health and helps your body function properly.

- **Small Frequent Meals:** Eating smaller meals throughout the day helps regulate blood sugar and provides your body with consistent energy.
- **Consider Fortified Foods:** Some foods are fortified with additional vitamins and minerals that can support your recovery.

Fueling Your Path to Recovery

By following these tips and focusing on a healthy diet, you can ensure your body receives the nutrients it needs to heal and recover after a stroke. Remember, good nutrition empowers you to regain your strength, improve your energy levels, and optimize your overall well-being on the road to recovery.

Swallowing Difficulties

Imagine a stroke affecting your ability to swallow safely and comfortably. It can be scary and frustrating. But the good news is, with the right support, you can overcome these swallowing difficulties, also known as dysphagia. This chapter will explore what dysphagia is, its symptoms, and strategies to help you regain safe swallowing after a stroke.

Understanding Dysphagia

Dysphagia is a difficulty swallowing food or liquids. After a stroke, damage to the brain areas controlling swallowing muscles can cause these difficulties. This can lead to:

- Coughing or choking during meals.
- Food or liquids going down the wrong pipe (aspiration).
- Feeling like food gets stuck in your throat.
- Drooling.
- Weight loss due to difficulty eating.

Recognizing the Signs

It is important to be aware of the signs of dysphagia after a stroke. Here are some things to watch for:

- Taking a long time to finish a meal.
- Difficulty chewing or controlling food in your mouth.
- Wet or hoarse voice after eating.

Getting Help for Dysphagia

If you suspect dysphagia after a stroke, it is important to seek medical attention right away. A doctor or speech-language pathologist (SLP) can assess your swallowing difficulties and recommend the best course of treatment.

Treatment Options for Dysphagia

There are different treatment options for dysphagia, depending on the severity of your condition:

- **Swallowing Exercises:** An SLP can teach you exercises to strengthen your swallowing muscles and improve coordination.
- **Dietary Modifications:** Your doctor or SLP might recommend specific food textures (thicker liquids, softer foods) to make swallowing safer.
- **Swallowing Techniques:** Learning special techniques like head positioning or holding your breath during swallowing can improve the process.
- **Thickening Liquids:** Adding thickeners to liquids can make them easier to swallow and prevent aspiration.

Living with Dysphagia

While dysphagia can be challenging, it does not have to control your life. Here are some tips for living well with dysphagia:

- **Work with your SLP:** Regular therapy sessions are crucial for improving swallowing skills.
- **Follow your doctor's recommendations:** Stick to the recommended diet and swallowing techniques.
- **Be patient:** Recovery takes time and effort. Celebrate even small improvements.
- **Maintain good oral hygiene:** This helps prevent infections that can worsen swallowing difficulties.
- **Talk to your family and friends:** Raising awareness about your condition can ensure they understand and support you during meals.

Remember: Dysphagia after stroke is manageable. By seeking medical attention, working with therapists, and making lifestyle adjustments, you can regain safe swallowing and enjoy eating again.

Creating a Safe and Healthy Eating Environment

Imagine recovering from a stroke and feeling nervous about mealtimes. But it does not have to be stressful. By creating a safe and healthy eating environment, you can enjoy meals with confidence and support your recovery journey. This chapter explores ways to make mealtimes safe, comfortable, and enjoyable after a stroke.

Safety First: Essential Considerations

After a stroke, swallowing difficulties (dysphagia) can be a concern. Here is how to prioritize safety during meals:

- **Seating:** Sit upright in a supportive chair with good back and neck support. This helps with posture and swallowing.
- **Minimize Distractions:** Turn off the TV or radio, and avoid conversations that require too much focus while eating.
- **Supervision:** If needed, have someone present to assist you during meals in case of choking or coughing.

Optimizing Your Comfort

Creating a comfortable environment makes eating more enjoyable and promotes better swallowing:

- **Pleasant Atmosphere:** Eat in a well-lit, calm, and relaxing space.
- **Adaptive Utensils:** Consider using weighted utensils for better grip, or specialized cups with spill-proof lids.
- **Comfortable Clothing:** Loose-fitting clothing allows for easier movement during meals.

Enhancing Your Enjoyment

Mealtimes shouldn't just be about safety; they can be a source of pleasure too. Here are some tips:

- **Presentation Matters:** Arrange food in an appealing way on a plate. Use colorful fruits and vegetables to brighten things up.
- **Involve Your Senses:** Notice the aroma, texture, and flavors of your food. Savor each bite.
- **Take Your Time:** Eat slowly and chew your food thoroughly. This aids digestion and helps prevent choking.
- **Socialize and Connect:** Share meals with loved ones whenever possible. Conversation can enhance the experience.

Working with Your Therapist:

Your speech-language pathologist (SLP) can be a valuable resource for creating a safe and healthy eating environment. They can:

- **Recommend adaptive equipment:** They can suggest specific utensils, plates, or cups that can make eating easier.
- **Offer swallowing strategies:** Your SLP might teach you special techniques to improve your swallowing safety and efficiency.
- **Provide guidance on food textures:** They can recommend the right food consistencies (thicker liquids, softer foods) based on your swallowing abilities.

Remember: Recovery is a journey, and mealtimes are an important part of it. By creating a safe, comfortable, and enjoyable eating environment, you can set yourself up for success during meals and support your overall well-being after a stroke.

Staying Hydrated

Imagine recovering from a stroke. You might feel weak, tired, and maybe even a little confused. Proper hydration, meaning getting enough fluids, is crucial for your recovery journey. This chapter explores why staying hydrated is so important after a stroke and offers tips for managing your fluid intake effectively.

Why is Hydration Important After Stroke?

Water makes up a major part of your body, and it plays a vital role in many functions:

- **Flushing Out Toxins:** Water helps your body eliminate waste products and keeps your system functioning smoothly.

- **Regulating Body Temperature:** Water helps you sweat and maintain a healthy body temperature, which is important after a stroke.
- **Delivering Nutrients:** Water transports essential nutrients to your cells throughout your body, supporting healing and recovery.
- **Aiding Digestion:** Water helps your digestive system function properly, preventing constipation, which can be a common problem after a stroke.
- **Boosting Energy Levels:** Dehydration can lead to fatigue and weakness. Staying hydrated keeps you alert and energized during recovery.

What Happens When You are Dehydrated?

Dehydration after a stroke can worsen your condition and lead to complications:

- **Thicker Blood:** Dehydration can thicken your blood, increasing the risk of blood clots, which can be dangerous after a stroke.
- **Kidney Problems:** Dehydration can put extra strain on your kidneys, which are already working hard to recover from the stroke.
- **Confusion:** Dehydration can lead to confusion and disorientation, making recovery more challenging.
- **Urinary Tract Infections (UTIs):** Dehydration can increase your risk of UTIs, which can be uncomfortable and require additional treatment.

How Much Fluid Do You Need?

The amount of fluid you need depends on various factors like your weight, activity level, and climate. A general guideline is to aim for eight glasses (or two liters) of water daily. However, it is best to talk to your doctor about the specific amount of fluid that's right for you after a stroke.

Tips for Staying Hydrated After Stroke

Here are some tips to ensure you get enough fluids after a stroke:

- **Carry a Water Bottle:** Keep a reusable water bottle with you throughout the day and take frequent sips.
- **Set Reminders:** Use alarms or phone notifications to remind yourself to drink water regularly.
- **Choose Your Beverages Wisely:** Water is best, but unsweetened tea, milk, and clear broths can also contribute to your fluid intake.
- **Make it Flavorful:** Add slices of lemon, cucumber, or berries to your water for a refreshing twist.
- **Eat Water-Rich Foods:** Fruits and vegetables like watermelon, celery, and tomatoes naturally contain high water content.
- **Monitor Your Urine:** Pale yellow urine indicates good hydration. Darker urine suggests dehydration.

Remember: Staying hydrated is an essential part of your recovery after a stroke. By following these tips and talking to your doctor, you can ensure you are getting the right amount of fluids to support your healing journey and feel your best.

Heart-Healthy Diet After Stroke

Imagine recovering from a stroke. You might feel a bit fragile and wonder what you can do to stay healthy. Well, good news. Eating a heart-healthy diet is like giving your heart a big hug after a scare. This chapter dives into the power of food choices and how they can support a strong heart and overall well-being after a stroke.

Why a Heart-Healthy Diet Matters After Stroke

Stroke often happens because of clogged arteries. These arteries supply blood to your brain, and when they're blocked, it can lead to stroke. A heart-healthy diet helps keep your arteries clear and reduces your risk of another stroke. But that's not all. It also helps with:

- **Lowering Blood Pressure:** High blood pressure puts extra stress on your heart and blood vessels. Eating a healthy diet can help keep your blood pressure in a healthy range.
- **Managing Cholesterol:** Certain foods can raise your bad cholesterol, which contributes to artery blockage. A heart-healthy diet keeps your cholesterol levels in check.
- **Maintaining a Healthy Weight:** Being overweight or obese increases your risk of stroke and heart disease. Eating healthy helps you maintain a healthy weight or lose weight if needed.

The Heart-Healthy All-Stars

So, what kind of food choices make your heart happy? Here are some key players in a heart-healthy diet:

- **Fruits and Vegetables:** These colorful wonders are packed with vitamins, minerals, and fiber, all essential for a healthy heart. Aim for at least five servings a day.
- **Whole Grains:** Whole grains like brown rice, quinoa, and whole-wheat bread provide sustained energy and fiber, which can help lower cholesterol.
- **Lean Protein:** Fish, chicken, beans, and lentils are great sources of protein for building and repairing tissues. Choose lean cuts of meat and limit processed meats.
- **Healthy Fats:** Do not ditch all fats. Healthy fats like those found in olive oil, avocado, and nuts are good for your heart.

- **Low-Fat Dairy:** Calcium-rich dairy products like yogurt and low-fat cheese are beneficial for bone health, but choose low-fat options to avoid added saturated fat.

Limiting the Troublemakers

Just like there are heart-healthy all-stars, there are some foods you might want to limit after a stroke:

- **Added Sugars and Sweets:** These can lead to weight gain and unhealthy blood sugar levels, putting a strain on your heart.
- **Saturated and Trans Fats:** These fats found in fried foods, processed meats, and pastries can increase your bad cholesterol and clog arteries.
- **Added Salt:** Too much salt can raise your blood pressure, which is not good for your heart.

Remember: A heart-healthy diet is a lifelong commitment, but it does not have to be complicated. Small changes add up.

Here are some additional tips:

- **Read Food Labels:** Pay attention to serving sizes, saturated and trans-fat content, and added sodium (salt) on food labels.
- **Cook More at Home:** This gives you more control over the ingredients and portion sizes in your meals.
- **Find Healthy Alternatives:** Swap fried foods for baked or grilled options. Choose water or unsweetened tea instead of sugary drinks.
- **Make it a Family Affair:** Involve your loved ones in planning and preparing healthy meals. Eating healthy together is a great way to support each other.

Fueling Your Recovery

By eating a heart-healthy diet after a stroke, you are not just protecting your heart; you are giving your body the best chance to heal and recover. With these delicious and nutritious choices, you can keep your heart happy and feel your best on the road to recovery. Remember, small changes can make a big difference.

Meal Planning and Preparation for Stroke Survivors

Imagine recovering from a stroke and feeling overwhelmed by the thought of cooking. But fear not. Meal planning and preparation can be a breeze with some clever strategies. This chapter empowers you, as a stroke survivor, to navigate the kitchen with confidence and enjoy delicious, healthy meals throughout your recovery journey.

Planning Makes Perfect: The Power of Meal Planning

Taking some time each week to plan your meals offers many benefits:

- **Saves Time and Energy:** Planning eliminates the daily scramble of "what's for dinner?" You will know exactly what you need to prepare, making cooking less stressful.
- **Promotes Healthy Choices:** Planning allows you to focus on incorporating heart-healthy and nutritious foods into your meals, supporting your recovery.
- **Reduces Food Waste:** By planning meals based on what you have or will buy, you will throw away less food, saving money and resources.
- **Budget-Friendly:** Planning helps you stick to your grocery budget by avoiding impulse purchases at the store.

Tips for Easy and Effective Meal Planning:

- **Consider Your Needs:** Focus on heart-healthy ingredients and choose textures that are easy to swallow if you have dysphagia (swallowing difficulties).
- **Involve Your Family:** Planning meals together can be a fun activity and ensure everyone enjoys the food choices.
- **Keep it Simple:** Opt for quick and easy recipes that do not require extensive prep time or complicated cooking techniques.
- **Plan Leftovers:** Cook double batches and enjoy leftovers for another meal, saving you time and energy.
- **Utilize Online Resources:** There are many websites and apps with stroke-friendly recipes to inspire your meal plans.

Prepping Like a Pro: Making Meal Prep Your Ally

Once you have your meal plan in place, meal prep can be a game-changer:

- **Chop Vegetables in Advance:** Wash and chop vegetables on the weekend so they're ready to use throughout the week.
- **Cook in Bulk:** Cook a large batch of grains like brown rice or quinoa to have a base ready for quick meals.
- **Portion Out Proteins:** Marinate and portion out proteins like chicken or fish for easy grilling or baking later.
- **Prepare Soups and Stews:** These hearty meals can be made ahead of time and reheat beautifully for convenient lunches or dinners.
- **Make Smoothies:** Freeze chopped fruits and vegetables for easy, nutritious smoothies packed with vitamins and minerals.

Remember: Meal prep does not have to be fancy or time-consuming. Even small steps like washing and chopping vegetables can save you precious time and energy during the week.

Kitchen Hacks for Stroke Survivors:

Here are some additional tips to make cooking easier and safer after a stroke:

- **Use Adaptive Equipment:** Consider tools like weighted utensils, easy-grip can openers, or raised cutting boards for better control and safety.
- **Simplify Recipes:** Do not be afraid to adapt recipes to your needs. Use pre-chopped vegetables or frozen ingredients to save time and effort.
- **Ask for Help:** Do not hesitate to ask family or friends for assistance with grocery shopping or certain cooking tasks.
- **Embrace New Technologies:** Explore slow cookers, instant pots, or other appliances that can simplify meal preparation.

More Than Just Food: The Joy of Cooking

Cooking can be a source of enjoyment and accomplishment, especially on your recovery journey. By planning your meals, prepping ingredients, and utilizing helpful tools, you can conquer the kitchen with confidence.

Remember, a healthy and delicious meal is just a few steps away. So, grab your apron, put on some music, and rediscover the joy of cooking nutritious and satisfying meals that support your recovery and well-being.

Nutritional Counseling for Stroke Survivors

Imagine recovering from a stroke. You might wonder what foods can help you heal and regain your strength. Nutritional counseling can be your compass, guiding you towards a personalized eating plan that supports your recovery journey. This chapter explores the benefits of nutritional counseling and how it can empower you, as a stroke survivor, to make informed choices about the food you eat.

Why Nutritional Counseling After Stroke?

Stroke can affect your body's ability to use nutrients effectively. A registered dietitian (RD), a specialized nutritionist, can provide invaluable guidance:

- **Understanding Your Needs:** An RD will assess your individual needs based on your stroke severity, swallowing abilities (dysphagia), and overall health.
- **Creating a Personalized Plan:** They will create a customized meal plan that incorporates heart-healthy foods, considers any dietary restrictions, and ensures you get the nutrients your body needs to heal.
- **Managing Dysphagia:** If you have swallowing difficulties, the RD can recommend appropriate food textures and thicknesses to make eating safe and enjoyable.
- **Setting Realistic Goals:** The RD will work with you to set achievable goals for healthy eating, weight management, and overall well-being.
- **Answering Your Questions:** They can address any concerns you have about food, nutrition, and how diet can support your recovery.

Benefits of Nutritional Counseling

Nutritional counseling offers a multitude of benefits for stroke survivors:

- **Improved Recovery:** A healthy diet provides the building blocks your body needs to repair damaged tissues and regain strength.

- **Reduced Risk of Future Strokes:** Eating a heart-healthy diet can help manage blood pressure, cholesterol, and weight, all of which are risk factors for stroke.
- **Enhanced Energy Levels:** Proper nutrition fuels your body for better energy throughout the day, helping you participate in rehabilitation activities.
- **Weight Management:** The RD can help you maintain a healthy weight, which is crucial for overall health after a stroke.
- **Improved Quality of Life:** Eating healthy can boost your mood and well-being, contributing to a better quality of life after stroke.

What to Expect During Nutritional Counseling

A typical session with an RD might involve:

- **Discussing Your Medical History:** The RD will review your medical history, stroke details, and any medications you are taking.
- **Assessing Your Dietary Habits:** They will ask about your current eating patterns, food preferences, and any challenges you face regarding food intake.
- **Developing a Personalized Plan:** Based on your assessment, the RD will create a tailored meal plan that aligns with your recovery needs and preferences.
- **Learning About Healthy Eating:** They will educate you on healthy food choices, portion control, and how to read food labels effectively.
- **Setting Goals and Tracking Progress:** You will work with the RD to set achievable goals and track your progress towards a healthier lifestyle.

Finding a Registered Dietitian

Many hospitals, rehabilitation centers, and outpatient clinics have registered dietitians on staff. You can also find RDs in private practice or through online resources.

Remember: Nutritional counseling is an ongoing partnership. Be open to communication and ask questions throughout your journey.

Making the Most of Nutritional Counseling

- **Come Prepared:** Write down any questions or specific concerns you have about your diet before your appointment.
- **Be Open and Honest:** Providing honest information about your eating habits and challenges allows the RD to create the most effective plan for you.
- **Actively Participate:** Ask questions, share your preferences, and express your concerns during your counseling sessions.
- **Follow the Plan:** Commit to following the personalized meal plan created by the RD for optimal results.
- **Celebrate Your Successes:** Acknowledge and reward yourself for achieving your dietary goals, no matter how small.

Your Roadmap to a Healthy Future

Nutritional counseling can be a powerful tool for stroke survivors. By working with a registered dietitian, you can chart a course towards a healthy and fulfilling life after stroke. Remember, the food you choose can significantly impact your recovery. With personalized guidance and dedicated effort, you can navigate the world of nutrition with confidence and pave the way for a healthier future.

6. EMOTIONAL AND MENTAL WELLBEING

Coping with Depression and Anxiety After Stroke

Imagine recovering from a stroke. You might feel relieved to be alive, but also overwhelmed by sadness or worry. It is normal. Stroke can affect your brain in ways that lead to depression and anxiety. This chapter explores these emotions and offers tools to help you cope and find your light again.

Why Do I Feel This Way?

Stroke can cause changes in the brain that affect your mood. Here is why you might be feeling down or anxious:

- **Brain Chemistry:** Stroke can disrupt brain chemicals that regulate mood, leading to depression or anxiety.
- **Loss of Function:** You might feel frustrated or sad if you are unable to do the things you used to enjoy due to stroke limitations.
- **Fear of the Future:** The uncertainty of recovery or the possibility of another stroke can trigger anxiety.
- **Loneliness and Isolation:** Stroke can make it harder to socialize, leading to feelings of loneliness and isolation, which can worsen depression and anxiety.

Recognizing the Signs

It is important to be aware of the signs of depression and anxiety after stroke:

- **Depression:** Feeling down, hopeless, or losing interest in activities you used to enjoy, changes in sleep or appetite, difficulty concentrating.

- **Anxiety:** Excessive worry, feeling on edge or restless, physical symptoms like rapid heartbeat or shortness of breath.

Do not Suffer in Silence: Seeking Help

If you are experiencing depression or anxiety after stroke, it is crucial to seek help. Here is what you can do:

- **Talk to Your Doctor:** Be open about your emotional state. They can assess your symptoms and recommend treatment options.
- **Consider Therapy:** Therapy can help you develop coping mechanisms for managing depression and anxiety.
- **Join a Support Group:** Connecting with other stroke survivors who understand your challenges can be very helpful.

Coping Strategies for Everyday Life

Here are some coping strategies you can use to manage depression and anxiety after stroke:

- **Stay Active:** Regular exercise, even mild activity, can improve mood and reduce anxiety.
- **Practice Relaxation Techniques:** Deep breathing, meditation, or mindfulness exercises can help calm your mind and body.
- **Maintain a Healthy Lifestyle:** Eat a balanced diet, get enough sleep, and find healthy ways to manage stress.
- **Connect with Loved Ones:** Social interaction and spending time with supportive people can boost your mood.
- **Engage in Activities You Enjoy:** Do things that bring you pleasure, even if you have to adapt them due to limitations.
- **Focus on Progress:** Celebrate small achievements in your recovery journey, no matter how big or small.

Remember: Recovery from stroke is a journey, not a destination. It is okay to feel down or anxious sometimes. With the right support and the tools, you learn, you can manage these emotions and find your way back to feeling hopeful and positive about the future.

Additional Tips:

- **Be Patient:** It takes time to heal emotionally after stroke. Be patient with yourself and celebrate small victories.
- **Set Realistic Goals:** Do not try to do too much too soon. Set achievable goals and adjust them as you progress.
- **Do not Be Afraid to Ask for Help:** Reach out to family, friends, or healthcare professionals for help when you need it.

Finding Your Light Again

While depression and anxiety are common after stroke, they do not have to define your life. With the right support, effective coping strategies, and a positive mindset, you can overcome these challenges and rediscover your joy and hope. Remember, there is light at the end of the tunnel. You are not alone on this journey.

Socialization and Support Groups

Imagine recovering from a stroke. You might feel isolated and wonder if you will ever connect with others again. The good news is, social interaction and support groups can be lifelines on your recovery journey. This chapter explores the importance of staying connected and how support groups can empower you to rebuild your social life after a stroke.

Why is Socialization Important After Stroke?

Stroke can impact your ability to communicate or move around, making social interaction challenging. But staying connected is crucial for several reasons:

- **Combats Loneliness and Isolation:** Social interaction helps you feel less alone and provides a sense of belonging.
- **Boosts Mood and Well-being:** Connecting with others can reduce stress, anxiety, and depression, promoting a more positive outlook.
- **Cognitive Stimulation:** Conversation and social activities can stimulate your brain, aiding cognitive recovery.
- **Provides Support and Encouragement:** Sharing experiences with others who understand your challenges can be incredibly motivating.
- **Improves Communication Skills:** Social interaction allows you to practice your communication skills in a safe and supportive environment.

Finding Your Tribe: The Benefits of Support Groups

Stroke support groups offer a unique space for connection and support:

- **Shared Experiences:** Connecting with other stroke survivors allows you to share experiences, challenges, and triumphs, fostering a sense of understanding.
- **Peer Support:** Learning from others who have faced similar situations can be incredibly motivating and provide valuable tips for your recovery.
- **Emotional Support:** Support groups offer a safe space to express your emotions and anxieties without judgment.
- **Information Sharing:** You can learn about resources, treatments, and coping strategies from other members and healthcare professionals.

- **Building Friendships:** Support groups can lead to lasting friendships with people who understand your journey.

Types of Support Groups

There are various support groups available:

- **In-Person Groups:** Meeting face-to-face allows for deeper connection and non-verbal communication.
- **Online Groups:** Online groups offer flexibility and access to a wider community, especially for those with mobility limitations.
- **Stroke-Specific Groups:** These groups focus on challenges and experiences specific to stroke survivors.
- **Family and Caregiver Groups:** Support groups exist for those who care for stroke survivors, offering guidance and emotional support.

Finding the Right Support Group

Here are some tips for finding the right support group for you:

- **Talk to Your Doctor:** They can recommend support groups in your area.
- **Consider Your Needs:** Choose a group that focuses on stroke or addresses specific challenges you face.
- **Research Online:** Many support groups have online presences where you can learn more about them.
- **Try Different Groups:** Do not be afraid to try different groups until you find one that feels like a good fit.

Remember: Taking the first step to join a support group can feel daunting, but it is worth it.

Making the Most of Support Groups

Here are some tips to get the most out of your support group experience:

- **Be Open and Share:** The more you share, the more you can connect with others and receive support.
- **Ask Questions:** Do not hesitate to ask questions and learn from others' experiences.
- **Listen and Offer Support:** Supporting others can also be a source of healing and connection.
- **Respect Boundaries:** Everyone's recovery journey is different. Be respectful of others' experiences and privacy.

Reconnecting with the World

Socialization and support groups can be powerful tools for rebuilding your social life after a stroke. By connecting with others who understand your journey, you can combat loneliness, boost your mood, and feel empowered on your path to recovery. Remember, you are not alone. So, take that first step, reach out, and rediscover the joy of connection and support.

Returning to Work or Daily Activities

Imagine recovering from a stroke and wondering if you will ever be able to work or do your usual activities again. The answer is yes. With dedication and planning, you can successfully return to your daily routine. This chapter explores the steps you can take to confidently navigate this important transition.

Assessing Your Readiness

Returning to work or daily activities depends on several factors:

- **Severity of Stroke:** The extent of your stroke will influence your physical and cognitive abilities.
- **Recovery Progress:** Your progress in rehabilitation plays a key role in determining your readiness to return to work or activities.
- **Your Occupation and Daily Life:** The demands of your work and daily activities will influence how you need to adapt.

Planning for a Smooth Transition

Here are some steps to ensure a smooth return to your routine:

- **Talk to Your Doctor:** They can assess your recovery progress and guide you on a safe return to work or activities.
- **Consider Occupational Therapy:** An occupational therapist can help you regain skills needed for work or daily activities and suggest adaptations if needed.
- **Communicate with Your Employer:** If returning to work, have an open conversation with your employer about your limitations and any modifications you might need.
- **Discuss Your Needs with Loved Ones:** Talk to family and friends about how they can support you as you return to your daily routine.

Making Adjustments for Success

Returning to work or activities might require some adjustments:

- **Gradual Return:** Consider a phased return to work, starting with fewer hours or modified duties.
- **Adaptive Equipment:** Utilize tools that can make tasks easier, like ergonomic keyboards or raised toilet seats.
- **Pacing Yourself:** Do not try to do too much too soon. Take breaks and listen to your body.

- **Ask for Help:** Do not be afraid to delegate tasks or ask for assistance when you need it.

Managing Fatigue

Fatigue is a common side effect after stroke. Here are some tips to manage it:

- **Schedule Breaks:** Plan rest periods throughout your day to prevent fatigue and maintain energy levels.
- **Prioritize Sleep:** Getting enough quality sleep is crucial for recovery and managing fatigue.
- **Manage Stress:** Stress can worsen fatigue. Practice relaxation techniques like deep breathing or meditation.

Finding the Balance

Finding the balance between work, activities, and rest is essential for successful recovery:

- **Listen to Your Body:** Pay attention to your energy levels and adjust your schedule accordingly.
- **Celebrate Small Victories:** Acknowledge your progress, no matter how small, to stay motivated.
- **Maintain a Positive Attitude:** A positive outlook can significantly enhance your recovery journey.

Remember: Returning to work or daily activities after a stroke takes time and patience. Do not be discouraged by setbacks. With careful planning, support from your healthcare team, and a positive attitude, you can successfully reintegrate into your routine and rediscover your sense of purpose and accomplishment.

Family Caregiver Support After Stroke

Imagine being a family caregiver for a loved one recovering from a stroke. It can be a rewarding experience, but also overwhelming. This chapter acknowledges the vital role you play and offers resources and strategies to support you throughout this journey.

The Unsung Heroes: The Importance of Family Caregivers

After a stroke, family members often step up as primary caregivers. Your role is crucial in supporting your loved one's physical and emotional well-being. Here is why your support matters:

- **Promoting Recovery:** Your encouragement, assistance with daily tasks, and emotional support can significantly impact your loved one's recovery.
- **Navigating the Healthcare System:** You might be responsible for appointments, medication management, and advocating for your loved one's needs.
- **Providing Emotional Support:** Being a pillar of strength and understanding can help your loved one cope with the emotional challenges of stroke.

The Weight of Responsibility: Recognizing the Challenges

Caregiving can be demanding, both physically and emotionally. Here are some potential challenges you might face:

- **Stress and Burnout:** The constant demands of caregiving can lead to stress, exhaustion, and feelings of burnout.
- **Balancing Responsibilities:** Juggling caregiving with work, family, and personal needs can be difficult.
- **Emotional Toll:** Witnessing your loved one's struggles can take an emotional toll.

Taking Care of Yourself: Essential Tips for Family Caregivers

To effectively care for your loved one, you need to take care of yourself too. Here are some essential tips:

- **Seek Support:** Do not be afraid to ask for help from family, friends, or respite care services.
- **Join a Support Group:** Connecting with other caregivers can offer valuable information, resources, and emotional support.
- **Prioritize Your Health:** Maintain healthy habits like good sleep, balanced meals, and regular exercise to manage stress and stay energized.
- **Set Boundaries:** It is okay to say "no" and set boundaries to avoid burnout. Delegate tasks and ask for help whenever possible.
- **Do not Forget Self-Care:** Schedule time for activities you enjoy, even if it is just a short break to read or relax.

Resources for Family Caregivers

There are many resources available to support you on your caregiving journey:

- **Stroke Association Websites:** Websites like the American Stroke Association (https://www.stroke.org/en/) and the Stroke Association (UK) (https://www.stroke.org.uk/) offer resources specifically for caregivers.
- **Support Groups:** Many hospitals, community centers, and online platforms offer support groups for caregivers.
- **Caregiver Training Programs:** Programs can equip you with skills and knowledge to manage your caregiving responsibilities effectively.
- **Mental Health Professionals:** Talking to a therapist can help you manage stress and cope with the emotional challenges of caregiving.

Remember: You are not alone. Caring for someone after a stroke is a noble act, but it is important to prioritize your own well-being. By seeking support, managing your stress, and taking care of yourself, you can be the best possible caregiver for your loved one.

Sexuality After Stroke

Imagine recovering from a stroke. You might wonder if intimacy will ever be the same. The good news is, a fulfilling sex life is possible after stroke. This chapter explores the impact of stroke on sexuality and offers tips for navigating intimacy with confidence.

Stroke and Sexuality: Understanding the Connection

Stroke can affect your physical and emotional well-being, impacting your sex life in various ways:

- **Physical Changes:** Stroke can lead to weakness, numbness, or difficulty with balance, affecting sexual function.
- **Fatigue:** Recovery can be tiring, leaving you with less energy for intimacy.
- **Emotional Challenges:** Depression, anxiety, or low self-esteem after stroke can affect your desire and enjoyment of sex.

Communication is Key

Talking openly and honestly with your partner is crucial:

- **Share Your Concerns:** Do not be afraid to express your anxieties or physical limitations regarding intimacy.
- **Listen to Your Partner:** Understand their needs and concerns as well.
- **Explore Together:** Be open to discussing different ways to find intimacy and pleasure.

Redefining Intimacy

Sexuality is about more than just intercourse. Here are ways to redefine intimacy after stroke:

- **Focus on Non-Sexual Touch:** Cuddle, hold hands, or give massages to create closeness and emotional connection.
- **Explore Sensuality:** Engage your senses with candles, music, or scented oils to create a romantic atmosphere.
- **Communication and Emotional Connection:** Talk, share feelings, and express affection verbally.

Making Adjustments

Depending on your specific limitations, you might need to make some adjustments:

- **Pacing Yourself:** Plan for intimacy when you have energy and schedule breaks if needed.
- **Explore Different Positions:** Find positions that are comfortable and safe for both of you.
- **Consider Assistive Devices:** Certain aids can help, like cushions for back support or lubricants for dryness.

Talking to Your Doctor

Do not hesitate to talk to your doctor about any problems you are experiencing with sexual function. They can:

- **Address Physical Concerns:** They might recommend medication or physical therapy to improve sexual function.
- **Refer You to a Specialist:** If needed, they can refer you to a specialist like a sex therapist for tailored guidance.

Remember: A healthy and fulfilling sex life is still possible after stroke. With open communication, patience, and a willingness to adapt, you and your partner can rediscover intimacy and emotional connection.

Here are some additional points to consider:

- **Be Patient:** Recovery takes time. Patience and understanding are key for both you and your partner.
- **Focus on Enjoyment:** The goal is to find ways to experience pleasure and connect with your partner, not necessarily perfect performance.
- **Seek Support:** Talk to a therapist or counselor if you are struggling with emotional or communication issues.

Sexuality is a beautiful part of life, and it can continue to be a source of joy and connection after stroke. With an open mind, effective communication, and a willingness to adapt, you can navigate intimacy with confidence and rediscover the pleasure of sharing love with your partner.

Fatigue Management

Imagine recovering from a stroke. You might feel like you can barely climb a flight of stairs without needing a nap. Fatigue, a feeling of extreme tiredness, is a common foe after stroke. But fear not, warrior. This chapter equips you with tools and strategies to manage fatigue and reclaim your energy on your recovery journey.

Why Do I Feel So Tired?

Stroke disrupts your brain's delicate balance, affecting your energy levels in several ways:

- **Brain Injury:** Healing from a stroke requires a lot of energy, leaving you feeling drained.
- **Medication:** Some medications used post-stroke can cause fatigue as a side effect.
- **Pain and Discomfort:** Pain and discomfort from injuries or limitations can disrupt your sleep and leave you feeling exhausted.
- **Emotional Stress:** Coping with the emotional challenges of stroke can be draining and contribute to fatigue.

The Effects of Fatigue

Fatigue can impact your recovery in several ways:

- **Hinders Rehabilitation:** Feeling constantly tired can make it harder to participate in physical or occupational therapy.
- **Increases Frustration:** Low energy levels can lead to frustration and negativity, hindering your progress.
- **Affects Mood:** Fatigue can worsen symptoms of depression and anxiety after stroke.
- **Decreases Quality of Life:** Constant tiredness can make it difficult to enjoy activities you used to love.

Taming the Fatigue Beast: Effective Strategies

Here is your battle plan for conquering fatigue:

- **Listen to Your Body:** Pay attention to your energy levels and schedule activities accordingly. Rest when you are tired, and do not push yourself too hard.
- **Pace Yourself:** Break down tasks into smaller, manageable chunks to avoid feeling overwhelmed.
- **Prioritize Sleep:** Aim for 7-8 hours of quality sleep each night. Develop a relaxing bedtime routine and create a sleep-conducive environment.

- **Exercise Regularly:** Regular, gentle exercise can improve your energy levels and sleep quality. Start with low-impact activities like walking or swimming.
- **Eat a Balanced Diet:** Nourish your body with healthy foods that provide sustained energy. Avoid sugary snacks that cause energy crashes.
- **Manage Stress:** Practice relaxation techniques like deep breathing or meditation to reduce stress and improve sleep.
- **Talk to Your Doctor:** If fatigue is severe or affecting your daily life, talk to your doctor. They can adjust medication or rule out underlying conditions.

Energy-Saving Tips for Daily Life

Here are some everyday tips to conserve your energy:

- **Delegate Tasks:** Do not be afraid to ask for help from family and friends with daily chores.
- **Use Assistive Devices:** Consider using canes, grab bars, or shower chairs to make daily tasks less tiring.
- **Simplify Activities:** Find easier ways to do things. For example, use a stool while washing dishes or cook in bulk to minimize cooking time.
- **Plan Your Day:** Schedule activities based on your energy levels. Save demanding tasks for when you feel most energetic.

Remember: Fatigue is a common challenge after stroke, but it can be managed with effective strategies. By listening to your body, prioritizing sleep, and making adjustments to your daily routine, you can reclaim your energy and continue your recovery journey feeling your best. You are not alone in this battle.

Building Self-Esteem and Confidence After Stroke

Imagine recovering from a stroke. You might feel a bit discouraged, wondering if you will ever feel like yourself again. But Here is the good news: you can rebuild your self-esteem and confidence after stroke. This chapter equips you with tools and strategies to rediscover your inner strength and approach your recovery with a positive outlook.

Why Does Stroke Affect My Confidence?

Stroke can impact your physical abilities, communication skills, or even the way you see yourself. These changes can lead to a dip in self-esteem and confidence. Here is why:

- **Loss of Independence:** Stroke might make you rely on others for daily tasks, which can affect your sense of self-reliance.
- **Frustration with Recovery:** The recovery process can be frustrating, leading to feelings of discouragement and self-doubt.
- **Changes in Appearance:** Stroke may cause some physical changes, which can negatively impact your self-image.

The Importance of Self-Esteem and Confidence

Strong self-esteem and confidence are crucial for a fulfilling life, especially after stroke. Here is how they can benefit you:

- **Motivation:** They fuel your motivation to participate in rehabilitation and reach your recovery goals.
- **Positive Thinking:** A positive outlook helps you cope with challenges and setbacks.
- **Resilience:** Self-esteem helps you bounce back from frustrations and stay focused on progress.
- **Improved Well-being:** Feeling good about yourself can enhance your mood and overall well-being.

Building Blocks of Confidence: Strategies for Success

Here are some key strategies to rebuild your self-esteem and confidence after stroke:

- **Focus on Progress, Not Perfection:** Celebrate small victories during your recovery, no matter how big or small. Each step forward is a win.
- **Set Realistic Goals:** Do not try to do too much too soon. Set achievable goals that motivate you and build a sense of accomplishment.
- **Focus on What You Can Control:** Focus on improving your abilities and the aspects of your life you can control.
- **Embrace Your New Normal:** Accept that things might be different after stroke, but that does not mean you cannot enjoy a fulfilling life.
- **Challenge Negative Thoughts:** Do not let negative self-talk discourage you. Challenge negative thoughts with positive affirmations about your strength and resilience.
- **Find Your Strengths:** Rediscover your talents and skills. Focus on what you are good at and find ways to incorporate those strengths into your life.
- **Connect with Others:** Surround yourself with supportive people who believe in you and celebrate your victories.
- **Celebrate Who You Are:** Remember, you are more than your stroke. Focus on your personality, values, and experiences that make you unique.

Remember: Building self-esteem and confidence takes time and effort. Be patient with yourself, celebrate your progress, and do not be afraid to seek additional support. Here are some resources that can help:

- **Talk Therapy:** Talking to a therapist can help you manage negative thoughts and develop coping mechanisms to boost your confidence.
- **Support Groups:** Connecting with others who understand your challenges can be a source of encouragement and inspiration.

Regaining Your Confidence: A Journey, Not a Destination

Rebuilding self-esteem and confidence after stroke is a journey, not a destination. By implementing these strategies, celebrating your victories, and surrounding yourself with supportive people, you can rediscover your inner strength and approach your recovery with a positive and confident mindset. You are braver than you believe, stronger than you seem, and smarter than you think.

Managing Anger and Frustration After Stroke

Imagine recovering from a stroke. You might feel frustrated with the slow progress, angry at the limitations, or upset with yourself. These emotions are completely normal. Stroke can be a life-changing event, and it is natural to experience anger and frustration along the way. This chapter equips you with tools to manage these emotions and navigate your recovery journey with a calmer mind.

Why Do I Feel This Way?

Stroke can lead to anger and frustration for several reasons:

- **Loss of Independence:** Relying on others for daily tasks can be frustrating, especially if you were previously independent.
- **Slow Recovery:** Healing takes time, and setbacks can be discouraging, leading to anger and impatience.
- **Changes in Communication:** Difficulty speaking or expressing yourself clearly can be frustrating and lead to outbursts.

- **Physical Limitations:** Inability to do the things you used to do can lead to a sense of helplessness and anger.
- **Brain Chemistry:** Stroke can disrupt brain chemicals that regulate mood, sometimes leading to increased anger or irritability.

The Dangers of Unmanaged Anger

Unmanaged anger can be harmful to you and those around you. Here is why it is important to manage your frustration:

- **Stress on Relationships:** Uncontrolled anger can strain relationships with loved ones and caregivers.
- **Increased Blood Pressure:** Anger can elevate your blood pressure, which is a risk factor for another stroke.
- **Hinders Recovery:** Constant frustration can make it harder to focus on rehabilitation and stay motivated.

Effective Strategies for Anger Management

Here are some strategies to manage anger and frustration after stroke:

- **Identify Your Triggers:** Recognize what situations or emotions trigger your anger. Once you know what sets you off, you can develop coping mechanisms.
- **Take Deep Breaths:** When you feel anger rising, take slow, deep breaths to calm your body and mind.
- **Count to Ten:** Counting to ten or using another calming technique can give you time to cool down before reacting.
- **Take a Time Out:** If you feel overwhelmed, excuse yourself from the situation and take a short break to calm down before returning.
- **Express Your Needs Assertively:** Learn to communicate your needs and frustrations assertively, without resorting to anger.

- **Practice Relaxation Techniques:** Techniques like meditation or progressive muscle relaxation can help manage stress and improve your overall well-being.
- **Talk to Your Doctor:** If you struggle to manage anger, talk to your doctor. They might recommend therapy or medication adjustments to help.

Finding Healthy Outlets for Frustration

Channeling your frustration into healthy outlets can be beneficial. Here are some ideas:

- **Exercise:** Regular physical activity is a great way to release frustration and improve your mood.
- **Hobbies and Activities:** Engage in activities you enjoy, like painting, listening to music, or spending time in nature.
- **Talk Therapy:** A therapist can help you develop coping mechanisms and communication skills to manage anger effectively.
- **Support Groups:** Connecting with others who understand your challenges can be a source of support and encouragement.

Remember: It is okay to feel angry or frustrated after stroke. These emotions are normal. The key is to develop healthy coping mechanisms to manage them effectively and prevent them from hindering your recovery.

Here are some additional tips:

- **Focus on Progress:** Celebrate your achievements, no matter how small, to boost your mood and reduce frustration.
- **Set Realistic Goals:** Unrealistic expectations can lead to disappointment and frustration. Set achievable goals and adjust them as needed.

- **Focus on What You Can Control:** Do not dwell on what you cannot control. Focus on improving your abilities and the aspects of your life you can influence.
- **Be Patient with Yourself:** Recovery takes time. Be patient, kind to yourself, and celebrate your victories along the way.

With a toolbox of strategies, a supportive environment, and a willingness to learn, you can gain control over your anger and frustration. Remember, you are not alone in this journey.

Spiritual Considerations After Stroke

Imagine recovering from a stroke. You might be questioning your place in the world, wondering if your faith or spirituality can offer comfort. The good news is, your spiritual journey can be a source of strength and solace after stroke. This chapter explores how spirituality can contribute to your recovery and offers ways to reconnect with your beliefs.

The Power of Spirituality After Stroke

Spirituality, broadly defined as a connection to something greater than yourself, can play a significant role in coping with stroke. Here is how:

- **Provides Comfort and Hope:** Spiritual beliefs can offer solace and a sense of purpose during challenging times.
- **Reduces Stress and Anxiety:** Focusing on faith or prayer can provide a sense of calm and reduce anxiety.
- **Promotes Strength and Resilience:** Spiritual practices can strengthen your inner resources to navigate the recovery journey.
- **Connects You to a Community:** Religious communities or spiritual groups can offer support, belonging, and a sense of shared purpose.

Exploring Your Spiritual Needs

Here are some questions to consider regarding your spiritual needs after stroke:

- Has your stroke affected your faith or beliefs?
- How can your spirituality contribute to your recovery?
- Are there specific religious practices or prayers that comfort you?
- Would you like to connect with a spiritual leader or faith community?

Rekindling Your Spiritual Connection

Whether you have always been religious or are now rediscovering your spirituality, here are ways to reconnect:

- **Prayer and Meditation:** Meditation or prayer can provide inner peace and a sense of connection to something larger than yourself.
- **Religious Practices:** Engage in practices that bring you comfort, like reading scripture, attending religious services, or performing rituals.
- **Spending Time in Nature:** Connecting with nature can be a spiritual experience, offering peace and a sense of renewal.
- **Helping Others:** Volunteering or helping others can be a source of meaning and spiritual fulfillment.
- **Finding Spiritual Guidance:** Talk to a spiritual leader, chaplain, or therapist who can offer support and guidance.

Remember:

- **There is No Right or Wrong Way:** Your spiritual journey is personal. Find practices that resonate with you and bring you comfort.

- **It is Okay to Question:** This is a natural part of the healing process. Talk to someone you trust about your doubts or fears.
- **Faith Can Be a Source of Strength:** Your spirituality can be a powerful tool for navigating the challenges of recovery.

Finding Your Light Again

While stroke can be a difficult experience, it can also be a catalyst for spiritual growth. By rediscovering your connection to something bigger than yourself, you can find strength, hope, and a renewed sense of purpose on your recovery journey.

Here are some additional points to consider:

- **Respecting Beliefs:** Respect the spiritual beliefs of others, even if they differ from your own.
- **Finding Support:** Support groups can be a source of inspiration and connection with others who share similar spiritual beliefs.
- **Gratitude:** Practicing gratitude for the good things in your life can boost your mood and improve your overall well-being.

The search for meaning and connection is a fundamental human need. By nurturing your spiritual well-being alongside your physical and emotional recovery, you can navigate your journey after stroke with greater strength and a brighter outlook on the future.

Body Image and Self-Perception After Stroke

Imagine recovering from a stroke. You might look in the mirror and see changes in your body. These changes, along with limitations you might experience, can affect how you see yourself. This chapter explores the concept of body image and self-perception after stroke, and offers ways to navigate these changes with acceptance and self-compassion.

The Mirror and You: Understanding Body Image

Body image is how you see your physical appearance and how you feel about your body. Stroke can impact body image in several ways:

- **Physical Changes:** Stroke might cause weakness, paralysis, or scarring, leading to feelings of dissatisfaction with your appearance.
- **Loss of Function:** Inability to perform certain activities due to stroke limitations can affect how you perceive your body's capabilities.
- **Comparison to Others:** Comparing yourself to others who haven't experienced stroke can lead to feelings of inadequacy.

The Impact on Self-Perception

Changes in body image can affect your overall self-perception, your sense of who you are. You might feel:

- **Less Confident:** Feeling self-conscious about your appearance can lead to a dip in self-confidence.
- **Frustration:** Limitations can be frustrating, impacting your self-esteem and sense of control.
- **Isolation:** You might withdraw from social activities due to body image concerns.

Strategies for Positive Self-Perception

Here are some strategies to cultivate a positive self-perception after stroke:

- **Focus on What You Can Control:** Instead of dwelling on limitations, focus on what your body can still do. Celebrate your achievements in rehabilitation.

- **Challenge Negative Thoughts:** Do not let negative self-talk define you. Challenge negativity with affirmations about your strength, resilience, and inner beauty.
- **Focus on Your Abilities:** Rediscover your skills and talents. Maybe you have developed new strengths during recovery. Celebrate those.
- **Embrace Your Uniqueness:** Everyone has a unique body with its own story. Your stroke is part of your story, but it does not define you.
- **Practice Self-Care:** Nourish your body with healthy foods and regular exercise. Get enough sleep and prioritize activities that bring you joy.
- **Connect with Others:** Surround yourself with supportive people who value you for who you are, not just your physical appearance.
- **Seek Professional Help:** If you struggle with body image issues, consider talking to a therapist who can help you develop healthy coping mechanisms.

Remember:

- **Healing Takes Time:** Adjusting to changes in your body and self-perception takes time. Be patient with yourself.
- **Focus on Progress:** Celebrate your progress, no matter how small. Each step forward is a victory.
- **You Are More Than Your Stroke:** Your stroke does not define you. You are a whole person with a unique story, experiences, and strengths.

Beauty Beyond the Surface

Recovery after stroke is about healing both your body and your mind. By focusing on your abilities, celebrating your progress, and surrounding yourself with love and support, you can cultivate a positive self-perception that goes beyond physical appearance.

Remember, your true beauty lies in your strength, resilience, and the amazing person you are inside and out.

Mindfulness and Relaxation Techniques for Stroke Recovery

Imagine recovering from a stroke. You might feel overwhelmed by stress, anxiety, and fatigue. But Here is the good news: mindfulness and relaxation techniques can be powerful tools to promote healing and improve your well-being after stroke. This chapter explores how these practices can help you manage stress, improve sleep, and navigate your recovery journey with greater peace of mind.

The Mind-Body Connection After Stroke

Stroke disrupts the delicate balance between your mind and body. Here is how:

- **Stress and Anxiety:** Coping with the aftermath of stroke can be stressful, leading to anxiety and tension.
- **Fatigue:** Stroke can cause fatigue, making it harder to relax and unwind.
- **Pain and Discomfort:** Pain and discomfort from injuries or limitations can disrupt sleep and increase stress.

The Power of Mindfulness and Relaxation

Mindfulness and relaxation techniques can be like a soothing balm for your mind and body:

- **Stress Reduction:** These practices can help calm your nervous system, reducing stress hormones and promoting relaxation.
- **Improved Sleep:** Relaxation techniques can improve your sleep quality, leaving you feeling more energized throughout the day.

- **Pain Management:** Mindfulness can help you manage pain by shifting your focus away from discomfort and promoting relaxation.
- **Enhanced Focus:** Relaxation techniques can improve your focus and concentration, which can be beneficial for rehabilitation exercises.

Techniques for Your Toolkit

Here are some easy-to-learn mindfulness and relaxation techniques you can incorporate into your daily routine:

- **Deep Breathing:** Take slow, deep breaths from your diaphragm. Focus on your breath, feeling your belly rise and fall with each inhalation and exhalation.
- **Progressive Muscle Relaxation:** Tense and release different muscle groups throughout your body, starting from your toes and working your way up. Focus on the feeling of relaxation spreading through your body.
- **Guided Meditation:** Listen to guided meditations that focus on relaxation, mindfulness, or positive imagery.
- **Visualization:** Imagine yourself in a peaceful place, focusing on the sights, sounds, and smells of that environment.
- **Mindful Movement:** Activities like gentle yoga or tai chi combine movement with mindfulness, promoting relaxation and body awareness.

Making Relaxation a Habit

Here are some tips to integrate mindfulness and relaxation into your daily life:

- **Schedule Relaxation Time:** Just like any other activity, schedule time for relaxation each day. Even 10-15 minutes can make a difference.
- **Create a Relaxing Environment:** Find a quiet, comfortable space where you can relax without distractions.
- **Be Patient:** Learning relaxation techniques takes practice. Be patient with yourself and do not get discouraged if you do not experience immediate results.
- **Find What Works for You:** Experiment with different techniques to find what works best for you.

Remember:

- **Mindfulness is a Skill:** The more you practice, the better you will become at managing stress and promoting relaxation.
- **Be Kind to Yourself:** Recovery is a journey, not a destination. Be patient and kind to yourself throughout the process.
- **Seek Support:** If you struggle with stress or anxiety, talk to your doctor or therapist. They can provide additional guidance and support.

Finding Your Inner Peace

Mindfulness and relaxation techniques are valuable tools for anyone, but especially for those recovering from stroke. By incorporating these practices into your daily routine, you can cultivate inner peace, manage stress, and promote overall well-being on your road to recovery. Remember, you are not alone on this journey. With dedication and self-compassion, you can find your calm and navigate your recovery with greater ease.

Art Therapy and Creative Expression After Stroke

Imagine recovering from a stroke. You might feel frustrated with limitations, struggling to express yourself the way you used to. But Here is the secret: art therapy can be a powerful tool for healing and creative expression after stroke. This chapter explores how art therapy can benefit your recovery and reignite your creative spark.

Beyond Words: The Power of Art Therapy

Art therapy is a form of therapy that uses creative expression to promote healing and well-being. Here is how it can be particularly helpful after stroke:

- **Non-Verbal Communication:** Stroke can sometimes affect your ability to communicate clearly. Art therapy provides an alternative way to express your thoughts, feelings, and experiences.
- **Improved Motor Skills:** Engaging in creative activities can improve hand-eye coordination, fine motor skills, and dexterity.
- **Stress Reduction:** Art therapy is a relaxing and enjoyable activity that can help manage stress and anxiety after stroke.
- **Boosted Confidence:** Creating art can be a source of accomplishment and pride, promoting self-esteem and confidence.
- **Emotional Processing:** Art therapy can provide a safe space to explore and express emotions related to your stroke experience.

Unleashing Your Inner Artist: No Experience Necessary.

The beauty of art therapy lies in its accessibility. Here is what you can expect:

- **No Artistic Expertise Needed:** This is not about creating masterpieces. It is about enjoying the creative process and expressing yourself freely.
- **Variety of Materials:** Art therapists use a wide range of materials like paints, clay, crayons, or even music and movement.

- **Focus on the Process:** The emphasis is on enjoying the creative journey, not the final product.

Beyond Therapy: The Power of Everyday Creativity

Art therapy can be a starting point, but you can also incorporate creative expression into your daily life:

- **Coloring Books:** Adult coloring books can be a relaxing and mindful activity.
- **Journaling:** Writing or drawing in a journal can help express your thoughts and feelings creatively.
- **Listening to Music:** Music can be a powerful mood booster and can also inspire creative expression through dance or movement.
- **Nature Walks:** Soaking in nature's beauty can spark creativity and provide a calming environment.

Remember:

- **Creativity is for Everyone:** Do not be afraid to experiment and explore different creative outlets.
- **Focus on Enjoyment:** The goal is to have fun and express yourself, not achieve perfection.
- **Celebrate Your Efforts:** Be proud of yourself for trying new things and expressing yourself creatively.

A World of Color and Possibility

Art therapy and creative expression can be a transformative experience after stroke. By exploring your creativity, you can improve your communication skills, manage stress, and rediscover a sense of joy and accomplishment. Remember, the journey of recovery is not just about physical healing, but also about emotional well-being and rediscovering your unique way of expressing yourself in the world. So, grab some paints, crayons, or simply take a walk-in nature, and let your creativity flow.

7. LONG-TERM CARE AND FUTURE PLANNING

Preventing Another Stroke

Imagine feeling strong and healthy after recovering from a stroke. You might wonder, "Can I prevent another one?" The good news is, yes. By adopting healthy habits and working with your doctor, you can significantly reduce your risk of experiencing another stroke. This chapter equips you with the knowledge and tools to take charge of your health and prevent future strokes.

Understanding Stroke Risk Factors

Several factors can increase your risk of stroke. Some you can control, while others cannot. Here are the key ones:

- **High Blood Pressure:** Uncontrolled high blood pressure is a major risk factor for stroke.
- **High Cholesterol:** High levels of bad cholesterol can contribute to stroke risk.
- **Diabetes:** Diabetes can damage blood vessels and increase stroke risk.
- **Smoking:** Smoking significantly increases your risk of stroke.
- **Atrial Fibrillation:** An irregular heartbeat can increase the risk of blood clots leading to stroke.
- **Obesity:** Being overweight or obese can contribute to high blood pressure and diabetes, increasing stroke risk.
- **Family History:** Having a family history of stroke puts you at a higher risk.

Taking Control of Your Health: Strategies for Prevention

While you cannot control everything, you can significantly reduce your risk of stroke by focusing on these key areas:

- **Healthy Diet:** Eat a balanced diet low in saturated fats, sodium, and added sugars. Focus on fruits, vegetables, whole grains, and lean protein sources.
- **Regular Exercise:** Aim for at least 30 minutes of moderate-intensity exercise most days of the week.
- **Maintain a Healthy Weight:** Losing weight if you are overweight or obese can significantly reduce your stroke risk.
- **Manage Blood Pressure:** Regularly monitor your blood pressure and work with your doctor to keep it under control.
- **Manage Cholesterol:** Get your cholesterol levels checked regularly and follow your doctor's recommendations to manage them.
- **Manage Diabetes:** If you have diabetes, work with your doctor to manage your blood sugar levels effectively.
- **Quit Smoking:** Smoking is a major risk factor. Quitting smoking significantly reduces your stroke risk.
- **Reduce Stress:** Chronic stress can increase your risk of stroke. Practice stress management techniques like meditation or yoga.
- **Medications:** Your doctor may prescribe medication to manage blood pressure, cholesterol, or other risk factors. Take them as directed.

Working with Your Doctor: A Partnership for Prevention

Your doctor is your partner in preventing another stroke. Here is what you can expect:

- **Regular Checkups:** Schedule regular checkups with your doctor to monitor your blood pressure, cholesterol, and other risk factors.
- **Open Communication:** Discuss your stroke risk factors and any concerns you may have with your doctor openly.
- **Following Your Doctor's Recommendations:** Trust your doctor's advice and follow their recommendations regarding medication, lifestyle changes, and follow-up appointments.

Remember:

- **Prevention is Key:** By adopting healthy habits and working with your doctor, you can significantly reduce your risk of another stroke.
- **Small Changes Make a Big Difference:** Even small changes to your lifestyle can have a positive impact on your stroke risk.
- **Empowerment Through Knowledge:** Educate yourself about stroke risk factors and prevention strategies to take charge of your health.

Taking Charge of Your Future

Preventing another stroke is an ongoing process, but it is definitely achievable with knowledge, commitment, and support. By prioritizing your health, making positive lifestyle changes, and working with your doctor, you can empower yourself to reduce your risk and enjoy a healthier, more fulfilling future.

Advanced Care Planning After Stroke

Imagine recovering from a stroke. You might wonder, "What if something happens again?" Advanced care planning is a crucial step in ensuring your wishes are respected if you are unable to make medical decisions for yourself. This chapter equips you with the knowledge and tools to have open conversations with loved ones and healthcare providers about your future care preferences.

Why is Advanced Care Planning Important After Stroke?

Stroke can sometimes leave lasting effects that may impact your ability to make medical decisions in the future. Here is why advanced care planning is crucial:

- **Ensures Your Wishes are Respected:** It allows you to communicate your preferences for medical treatment in case you cannot speak for yourself.
- **Reduces Stress for Loved Ones:** Difficult medical decisions become easier for your family if they know your wishes beforehand.
- **Promotes Open Communication:** Planning facilitates important conversations about your values and beliefs regarding healthcare.

What Does Advanced Care Planning Involve?

Advanced care planning involves several key documents and discussions:

- **Durable Power of Attorney for Healthcare:** This document appoints someone you trust to make medical decisions if you cannot.
- **Living Will (Advance Directive):** This document outlines your wishes for treatment, such as life support or pain management.
- **Conversations with Loved Ones and Healthcare Providers:** Open communication is crucial to ensure everyone understands your wishes.

Having "The Talk" - Approaching Conversations About Your Care

Talking about your healthcare preferences can be difficult. Here are some tips for approaching these conversations:

- **Choose the Right Time:** Pick a calm and relaxed time when everyone feels comfortable.
- **Start Early:** Do not wait until a crisis to initiate these discussions.

- **Be Clear and Specific:** Clearly state your wishes regarding medical treatments you want or do not want.
- **Express Your Values:** Talk about what matters most to you in your care, quality of life, or pain management.
- **Update Regularly:** Review and update your documents as your health or preferences change.

Remember:

- **This is Your Decision:** You have the right to make choices about your healthcare.
- **It is Okay to Change Your Mind:** Your preferences can evolve over time. Update your documents accordingly.
- **Planning Brings Peace of Mind:** Having your wishes documented gives you and your loved ones peace of mind about your future care.

Planning for a Secure Future

Advanced care planning may seem daunting, but it is an important step towards a secure future. By having open conversations, documenting your wishes, and appointing someone you trust, you can ensure your values and preferences guide your care even if you cannot speak for yourself. Remember, open communication with loved ones and healthcare providers is key. Having a plan brings peace of mind to you and your family, allowing you to focus on your recovery with a sense of control and confidence.

Financial Considerations After Stroke

Imagine recovering from a stroke. You might be worried about medical bills, lost income, and how to manage your finances moving forward. This chapter addresses these concerns and equips you with tools to navigate the financial landscape after stroke.

The Financial Impact of Stroke

Stroke can be a significant financial burden. Here is why:

- **Medical Expenses:** Hospital stays, rehabilitation, medications, and ongoing care can be costly.
- **Loss of Income:** Stroke may limit your ability to work, impacting your financial security.
- **Increased Dependence on Others:** You might need help with daily tasks, leading to additional expenses for home care or modifications.

Planning and Preparation: Taking Control of Your Finances

Here are some strategies to manage your finances after stroke:

- **Gather Information:** Collect all your medical bills, insurance information, and employment details.
- **Review Insurance Coverage:** Understand your health and disability insurance plans and how they can help.
- **Explore Government Benefits:** Research government programs that might offer financial assistance for stroke survivors.
- **Talk to Your Employer:** Discuss options for returning to work or accessing disability leave.
- **Create a Budget:** Track your income and expenses to see where your money goes and identify areas for saving.
- **Seek Financial Assistance:** There might be organizations or programs offering financial support for stroke survivors.

Managing the Costs of Care

Here are some tips for managing medical bills and other care-related expenses:

- **Negotiate with Hospitals and Providers:** Do not be afraid to negotiate medical bills and explore payment plans.
- **Research Medical Equipment Costs:** Compare prices of medical equipment needed at home.
- **Consider Cost-Saving Alternatives:** Look for cost-effective options for medication, transportation, or home care.
- **Apply for Financial Aid Programs:** Hospitals and charities might offer financial aid programs for qualified patients.

Looking Ahead: Securing Your Financial Future

Here are some steps to secure your financial future after stroke:

- **Disability Insurance:** Consider disability insurance to provide income if you are unable to work.
- **Long-Term Care Planning:** Explore long-term care options and their associated costs.
- **Review Estate Planning:** Make sure your will and power of attorney are up-to-date.
- **Seek Financial Advice:** Consult a financial advisor who specializes in cases like stroke recovery.

Remember:

- **You are Not Alone:** Many resources are available to help you manage the financial impact of stroke.
- **Communication is Key:** Talk openly with healthcare providers, social workers, and financial advisors to explore your options.
- **Empowerment Through Knowledge:** Educate yourself about financial resources and benefits available to stroke survivors.

Financial security is a crucial concern after stroke. By taking a proactive approach, gathering information, exploring your options, and seeking financial guidance, you can navigate the financial complexities of recovery with greater peace of mind. Remember, there are resources available to help. With planning and careful management, you can secure a financially stable future for yourself and your loved ones.

Finding Your Support System

Imagine recovering from a stroke. You might feel overwhelmed and unsure where to turn for help. The good news is, you do not have to navigate this journey alone. This chapter explores a wealth of resources and support organizations available to stroke survivors, empowering you to connect with the help you need to thrive after stroke.

Building Your Support Network: Why It Matters

A strong support system is crucial for a successful stroke recovery. Here is why:

- **Emotional Support:** Support groups and counselors can provide a safe space to share your experiences and connect with others who understand your challenges.
- **Information and Resources:** Support organizations offer valuable information about stroke recovery, rehabilitation options, and available benefits.
- **Motivation and Encouragement:** Connecting with others who have overcome similar challenges can boost your motivation and provide hope for your recovery.

A World of Resources at Your Fingertips

Here are some key resources available for stroke survivors:

- **Stroke Support Groups:** Connecting with other survivors can provide emotional support and a sense of belonging.

- **Rehabilitation Centers:** These facilities offer specialized programs to help you regain your physical, cognitive, and emotional skills.
- **Government Agencies:** Government agencies like Social Security might offer financial assistance and support programs.
- **Charities and Non-Profit Organizations:** Many charities and non-profit organizations offer resources, equipment loans, and financial assistance to stroke survivors.
- **Online Resources:** Websites and online communities offer information, support groups, and educational materials about stroke recovery.

Finding the Right Support for You

With so many options, Here is how to find the support that fits your needs:

- **Talk to Your Doctor:** Your doctor can connect you with local support groups, rehabilitation centers, and other resources.
- **Search Online:** Use search engines or websites of stroke organizations to find support groups or resources in your area.
- **Consider Your Needs:** Choose a support group that focuses on specific challenges you face, like aphasia or communication difficulties.
- **Do not Be Afraid to Try Different Options:** Find a support group or resource that feels comfortable and helpful for you.

The Power of Advocacy

Stroke organizations also play a vital role in advocating for stroke survivors. They work to:

- **Increase Awareness:** Raise public awareness about stroke prevention and risk factors.

- **Fund Research:** Support research to improve stroke treatment and recovery options.
- **Lobby for Policy Changes:** Advocate for policies that improve access to stroke care and support for survivors.

Remember:

- **Help is Available:** You do not have to face recovery alone. There are many resources and support organizations available to help you.
- **There is Strength in Numbers:** Connecting with others who understand your journey can be incredibly empowering.
- **Be Your Own Advocate:** Do not hesitate to reach out for the support you need to optimize your recovery and live a fulfilling life after stroke.

Finding the right support system is essential for stroke recovery. By utilizing the resources available, connecting with support groups, and advocating for your needs, you can build a strong network that empowers you to reach your full potential and thrive after stroke. Remember, there is hope, and there is help. With knowledge, support, and a positive attitude, you can navigate your recovery with confidence and build a bright future for yourself.

Legal and Ethical Considerations After Stroke

Imagine recovering from a stroke. You might wonder about your rights, legalities surrounding your care, and how to make informed decisions. This chapter explores legal and ethical considerations after stroke, empowering you to navigate your healthcare journey with confidence.

Understanding Your Rights

After a stroke, you have certain legal rights as a patient. Here is what you need to know:

- **Right to Informed Consent:** You have the right to understand your medical condition, treatment options, and potential risks before consenting to any procedures.
- **Right to Refuse Treatment:** You have the right to refuse any treatment, even if it is recommended by your doctor.
- **Right to Privacy:** Your medical records are confidential, and you have control over who has access to them.
- **Right to Choose Your Care Provider:** You have the right to choose the doctor or healthcare facility that provides your care.

Making Decisions When You Cannot: Advanced Directives

Stroke can sometimes affect your ability to make medical decisions in the future. Here is where advanced directives come in:

- **Durable Power of Attorney for Healthcare:** This legal document appoints someone you trust to make medical decisions on your behalf if you cannot.
- **Living Will (Advance Directive):** This document outlines your wishes for treatment, such as life support or pain management, in case you cannot speak for yourself.

Ethical Considerations in Your Care

Ethical dilemmas can sometimes arise during healthcare. Here are some points to consider:

- **Quality of Life vs. Life Extension:** Discussions about life support and treatment options should focus on your values and desired quality of life.

- **Rationing of Care:** In rare cases, resources might be limited. You have the right to understand how decisions about care are made.
- **End-of-Life Care:** Open communication with your doctor and loved ones regarding your wishes for end-of-life care is crucial.

Advocating for Yourself and Others

Here are some tips for advocating for yourself and others:

- **Ask Questions:** Do not hesitate to ask questions and clarify any doubts you have about your care.
- **Express Your Wishes Clearly:** Communicate your preferences for treatment openly with your doctor and family.
- **Seek Support from Advocates:** Patient advocacy organizations can provide guidance and support in navigating healthcare decisions.

Remember:

- **Knowledge is Power:** Educating yourself about your rights and legal options empowers you to make informed decisions about your care.
- **Communication is Key:** Open communication with your doctor, family, and healthcare providers ensures your wishes are respected.
- **You Have a Voice:** Do not be afraid to advocate for yourself and ensure you receive the care you deserve.

Recovery is a Journey, Not a Destination

The legal and ethical considerations after stroke can seem complex, but with knowledge and open communication, you can navigate your healthcare journey with confidence. Remember, you have rights as a patient, and your voice matters. By advocating for yourself and understanding the ethical considerations surrounding your care, you can ensure your recovery journey is guided by your values and empowers you to live a fulfilling life after stroke.

End-of-Life Care Considerations After Stroke

Imagine recovering from a stroke. You might wonder, "What if things do not get better?" End-of-life care considerations may seem difficult to discuss, but planning for the future ensures your wishes are respected, and your loved ones are prepared. This chapter explores the importance of end-of-life care planning after stroke and guides you through making informed decisions about your care at the end of life.

Why is End-of-Life Care Planning Important After Stroke?

Stroke can sometimes impact your long-term health. Here is why end-of-life care planning is crucial:

- **Ensuring Your Wishes are Respected:** It allows you to communicate your preferences for comfort care and pain management at the end of life.
- **Reducing Stress for Loved Ones:** Difficult decisions become easier for your family if they know your wishes beforehand.
- **Promoting Open Communication:** Planning facilitates important conversations about your values and beliefs regarding end-of-life care.

What Does End-of-Life Care Planning Involve?

End-of-Life care planning involves several key considerations:

- **Discussing Your Values:** Talk to loved ones about what matters most to you at the end of life - comfort, pain management, or spending time with family.
- **Completing Advance Directives:** Living Wills and Durable Power of Attorney for Healthcare documents outline your wishes for care and appoint someone you trust to make decisions on your behalf if you cannot.
- **Understanding Palliative Care:** This specialized care focuses on comfort and managing pain at the end of life, regardless of diagnosis or prognosis.
- **Hospice Care:** Hospice care provides comfort and support for terminally ill patients and their families in a home setting or hospice facility.

Having "The Talk" - Approaching Conversations About Your Care

Talking about end-of-life care can be difficult. Here are some tips for initiating these conversations:

- **Choose the Right Time:** Pick a calm and relaxed time when everyone feels comfortable.
- **Start Early:** Do not wait until a crisis to initiate these discussions.
- **Be Open and Honest:** Express your wishes and fears openly with your loved ones.
- **Listen to Their Concerns:** Be open to your family's concerns and feelings about your wishes.
- **Review Regularly:** Update your documents and revisit these conversations as your health or preferences change.

Remember:

- **This is Your Decision:** You have the right to make choices about your end-of-life care.

- **It is Okay to Change Your Mind:** Your preferences can evolve over time. Update your documents accordingly.
- **Planning Brings Peace of Mind:** Having your wishes documented gives you and your loved ones peace of mind about your future care.

Facing the Future with Dignity

End-of-life care planning after stroke is about preparing for the future with dignity and ensuring your wishes are respected. By having open conversations, documenting your preferences, and exploring hospice or palliative care options, you can empower your loved ones to support you during this sensitive time. Remember, open communication is key. Planning for the future allows you to focus on living a fulfilling life in the present, knowing your wishes will be honored when the time comes.

Living Well with a Long-Term Disability After Stroke

Imagine recovering from a stroke, but things are not quite the same. Living with a long-term disability can be challenging, but it does not have to define you. This chapter explores strategies and tips for living a full and meaningful life after a stroke, even with limitations.

Adjusting to a New Normal

Coming to terms with a long-term disability can be difficult. Here is how to navigate the initial adjustment:

- **Allow Yourself to Grieve:** It is normal to feel sad, angry, or frustrated about the changes. Acknowledge your emotions and allow yourself time to heal.
- **Focus on What You Can Do:** Instead of dwelling on what you cannot do, shift your focus towards activities you can still enjoy and excel at.

- **Accept Support:** Do not be afraid to ask for help from family, friends, or healthcare professionals.

Living a Fulfilling Life with a Disability

Living well with a disability is possible. Here are some key strategies:

- **Set Realistic Goals:** Break down large goals into smaller, achievable steps. Celebrate your progress, no matter how small.
- **Explore Adaptive Technologies:** Assistive devices and technology can make daily tasks easier and help you live more independently.
- **Stay Active:** Physical activity is crucial for both physical and mental health. Find activities you can enjoy, like swimming or yoga.
- **Connect with Others:** Social interaction is vital. Join support groups, connect with friends, or volunteer in your community.
- **Maintain a Positive Attitude:** A positive outlook can make a world of difference. Focus on the things you can control and celebrate your resilience.

Making the Most of Your Life

Here are some additional tips for thriving with a disability:

- **Advocate for Yourself:** Do not be afraid to speak up for your needs and access to resources.
- **Educate Others:** Help others understand your disability and how they can best support you.
- **Focus on Your Passions:** Pursue hobbies or interests that bring you joy and a sense of purpose.
- **Find Inspiration:** Connect with stories of others who have overcome challenges to live fulfilling lives.

Remember:

- **You Are Not Alone:** Many people live well with long-term disabilities.
- **You Are Still You:** Your disability does not define you. It is just a part of your story.
- **Life Can Be Beautiful:** With the right mindset and support, you can still live a full and meaningful life after a stroke.

Living with a long-term disability is a journey, not a destination. By embracing change, seeking support, and focusing on what matters most to you, you can navigate this journey with strength and resilience. Remember, you are capable of living a life filled with joy, purpose, and endless possibilities.

Living with Aphasia in the Long Term

Imagine recovering from a stroke, but the words you once knew seem lost. Living with aphasia, a communication disorder caused by stroke, can be isolating and frustrating. But this chapter offers hope. Here, we will explore strategies and support systems to help you communicate effectively and live a fulfilling life after stroke, even with aphasia.

Understanding Aphasia: A Spectrum of Communication Challenges

Aphasia affects everyone differently. Here is a breakdown of some key types:

- **Expressive Aphasia:** Difficulty finding the right words to express yourself.
- **Receptive Aphasia:** Trouble understanding spoken language.
- **Anomic Aphasia:** Forgetting the names of objects or people.

Learning to Communicate in New Ways

While aphasia can be challenging, there are ways to overcome communication barriers:

- **Speech Therapy:** Working with a speech-language pathologist can help you regain lost skills and develop new communication strategies.
- **Augmentative and Alternative Communication (AAC):** Using tools like picture boards, apps, or electronic devices to communicate.
- **Nonverbal Communication:** Gestures, facial expressions, and drawing can be powerful ways to express yourself.
- **Patience and Practice:** Recovery takes time and effort. Be patient with yourself and celebrate your progress.

Living a Rich and Connected Life with Aphasia

Here are some tips for thriving despite aphasia:

- **Join a Support Group:** Connecting with others who understand your challenges can be incredibly helpful.
- **Find Activities You Enjoy:** Pursue hobbies or interests that do not rely heavily on spoken language, like art, music, or nature walks.
- **Stay Social:** Do not isolate yourself. Friends and family can learn new ways to communicate with you.
- **Advocate for Yourself:** Let others know how they can best support you in communication.
- **Technology Can Help:** Explore assistive technologies like voice recognition software or communication apps.

Remember:

- **Aphasia Does not Define You:** You are still the same intelligent and capable person you were before.
- **Communication is Still Possible:** There are many ways to connect with others, even with aphasia.
- **There is Hope:** With dedication and support, you can continue to learn, grow, and live a fulfilling life.

Living with aphasia in the long term requires resilience and a positive attitude. By embracing new communication methods, seeking support, and focusing on your strengths, you can rediscover your voice and build a life filled with connection and meaning. Remember, you are not alone on this journey. There are resources and people who can help you thrive despite the challenges of aphasia.

Advance Directives and Power of Attorney

Imagine yourself after a medical event, unable to speak for yourself. Who would make important decisions about your care? Advance directives and power of attorney documents ensure your wishes are respected, even when you cannot express them directly. This chapter explains these crucial tools for planning your future healthcare.

Making Your Voice Heard: What are Advance Directives?

Advance directives are legal documents that outline your preferences for medical treatment in case you become unable to make decisions for yourself due to illness or injury. Here are the two main types:

- **Living Will:** This document specifies your wishes regarding life-sustaining treatments like CPR or mechanical ventilation. You can choose to accept or refuse these interventions under certain circumstances.

- **Durable Power of Attorney for Healthcare:** This document appoints a trusted person (your "healthcare agent") to make medical decisions on your behalf if you cannot. You can give your agent broad authority or specific instructions.

Choosing Your Healthcare Hero: Power of Attorney Explained

A durable power of attorney for healthcare is like giving someone a key to your healthcare wishes. Here is what it means:

- **Your Trusted Agent:** Choose a reliable and responsible person who understands your values and beliefs about healthcare. Discuss your preferences with them openly.
- **Decision-Making Authority:** Your agent can make various decisions, from authorizing treatments to consenting to procedures, based on your wishes and best interests.
- **Your Right to Change Your Mind:** You can revoke or change your power of attorney document at any time as long as you are mentally competent.

Benefits of Advance Directives and Power of Attorney

Having these documents in place offers several advantages:

- **Peace of Mind:** Knowing your wishes are documented gives you and your loved ones peace of mind.
- **Reduced Family Stress:** During a difficult time, your family won't have to guess your wishes for care.
- **Respecting Your Choices:** Healthcare providers will honor your preferences as documented in advance directives.

Having "The Talk" - Discussing Your Wishes

Talking about healthcare decisions can be uncomfortable. Here are some tips:

- **Choose the Right Time:** Pick a calm and relaxed moment when everyone feels comfortable.
- **Open Communication:** Talk openly about your values and preferences regarding medical treatment.
- **Educate Yourself:** Learn about different treatment options before making decisions.
- **Ask Questions:** Do not hesitate to ask your doctor for clarification on any medical terms or procedures.

Remember:

- **This is Your Decision:** You have the right to choose the kind of care you want and to appoint someone you trust to make decisions on your behalf.
- **Planning is Key:** Do not wait until a crisis to create these documents.
- **Keep it Up-to-Date:** Review and update your advance directives and power of attorney as your health or preferences change.

Taking Control of Your Healthcare Future

Advance directives and power of attorney empower you to plan for your future healthcare. By creating these documents and having open conversations with loved ones and healthcare providers, you ensure your wishes are respected, even if you cannot speak for yourself. Remember, it is about taking control and ensuring your voice is heard, even when you cannot speak.

Housing Modifications for Accessibility After Stroke

Imagine returning home after a stroke. You might find familiar spaces suddenly feel challenging. But fear not. This chapter explores housing modifications that can transform your home into a safe, comfortable, and accessible haven, promoting your independence after stroke.

Why Modify Your Home?

Stroke can sometimes impact your mobility and balance. Here is how modifications can help:

- **Increased Safety:** Modifications can prevent falls and accidents, promoting safe living.
- **Improved Independence:** Changes can make daily tasks easier, allowing you to stay independent for longer.
- **Enhanced Comfort:** A comfortable and accessible home fosters your well-being and recovery.

Modifications for Everyday Living

Here are some key areas to consider for modifications:

- **Bathroom:** Grab bars in the shower or bathtub, a raised toilet seat, and slip-resistant flooring can increase safety.
- **Kitchen:** Lower cabinets, easy-grip handles, and pull-out shelves can make cooking and reaching items easier.
- **Living Areas:** Wider doorways, ramps instead of stairs, and good lighting can improve mobility and navigation.
- **Bedroom:** A raised bed, grab bars near the bed, and handrails in hallways can enhance safety and independence.

Finding the Right Modifications

Here are some tips for choosing the right modifications:

- **Occupational Therapist Evaluation:** An occupational therapist can assess your needs and recommend specific modifications.

- **Consider Your Needs:** Choose modifications that address your current and anticipated future needs.
- **Think Long-Term:** Opt for adaptable features that can be adjusted as your needs evolve.
- **Financial Considerations:** Explore options like grants, loans, or insurance coverage that might help with modification costs.

Making Your Home Accessible Does not Have to Be Expensive

Here are some ideas for budget-friendly modifications:

- **Install grab bars strategically** in bathrooms and hallways for added support.
- **Add raised toilet seats** for easier sitting and standing.
- **Rearrange furniture** to create wider, more navigable pathways.
- **Improve lighting** to increase visibility and prevent falls.
- **Use non-slip mats** in the bathroom and kitchen to prevent slipping.

Remember:

- **A Little Goes a Long Way:** Even small modifications can significantly improve accessibility in your home.
- **Safety First:** Prioritize modifications that enhance safety and prevent falls.
- **There are Options for Everyone:** Solutions exist to fit your needs and budget.

Creating an Accessible Oasis

Housing modifications are an investment in your well-being. By making your home safe, comfortable, and accessible, you can regain your independence and enjoy a better quality of life after stroke. Remember, with a few adjustments, your home can transform into a haven that supports your recovery journey and empowers you to live life to the fullest.

Government Assistance Programs for Stroke Survivors

Imagine recovering from a stroke. You might be worried about finances, healthcare access, and additional support. The good news is, many governments offer assistance programs to help stroke survivors navigate their recovery journey. This chapter explores some common types of government programs available in many countries.

Why are Government Assistance Programs Important?

Stroke can be a significant financial and social burden. These programs can help by:

- **Reducing Medical Costs:** Programs may offer financial assistance with medical bills, medication, and rehabilitation services.
- **Providing In-Home Care:** Some programs offer support for in-home care services, allowing you to stay independent for longer.
- **Offering Disability Benefits:** Financial assistance may be available for stroke survivors with long-term disabilities.
- **Supporting Employment:** Programs might offer help with job retraining or vocational rehabilitation to re-enter the workforce.
- **Connecting You to Resources:** Government agencies can connect you with support groups, counseling services, and other valuable resources.

Types of Government Assistance Programs

Here is a breakdown of some common programs offered by governments:

- **Social Security or Disability Benefits:** These programs provide financial assistance to individuals with disabilities, including stroke survivors who are unable to work.
- **Medicare/Medicaid (US) or National Health Services (UK):** These government-funded health insurance programs can help cover the costs of stroke treatment, rehabilitation, and ongoing medical care.
- **Home Care Services:** Some programs provide financial assistance or subsidized services for in-home care, such as bathing, dressing, and meal preparation.
- **Vocational Rehabilitation:** These programs offer training and support to help stroke survivors regain job skills and re-enter the workforce.
- **Transportation Assistance:** Programs may offer subsidized transportation services for doctor appointments, therapy sessions, or errands.

Eligibility and Applying for Assistance

Eligibility for these programs varies by country and individual circumstances. Here is what you need to know:

- **Contact Your Local Government Agency:** They can provide information on available programs and eligibility requirements.
- **Gather Documentation:** You might need medical records, proof of income, and other documents to apply.
- **Seek Help from Social Workers:** Hospitals or social workers can guide you through the application process.

Remember:

- **Help is Available:** Do not hesitate to explore government assistance programs that can ease your financial burden and support your recovery.

- **Programs Vary by Country:** Research specific programs offered by your government.
- **Seek Guidance:** Do not be afraid to ask for help from social workers or government agencies in navigating the application process.

Government Assistance: A Stepping Stone to Recovery

Government assistance programs play a crucial role in supporting stroke survivors on their road to recovery. These programs can offer financial relief, access to essential services, and resources to help you live a more independent and fulfilling life after stroke. Remember, you do not have to navigate this journey alone. By exploring available programs and seeking guidance, you can access the support you deserve to rebuild your life.

8. THE STROKE JOURNEY: STORIES OF RESILIENCE

Voices of Stroke Survivors and Caregivers

Imagine recovering from a stroke. You might feel overwhelmed and wonder, "Am I alone in this?" This chapter shares inspiring stories from stroke survivors and caregivers, offering encouragement, hope, and a sense of community on your recovery journey.

A Stroke Does not Define You: Sarah's Story

Sarah, a vibrant artist, suffered a stroke at the young age of 35. Her right arm was paralyzed, and she struggled to speak clearly. Devastated, she withdrew from her art and social life. But with therapy and unwavering support from her family, Sarah began to paint again, using her left hand. Today, she creates beautiful abstract pieces, her art reflecting her resilience and journey. "Stroke changed me," Sarah says, "but it didn't define me. I found a new way to express myself, and I'm stronger than ever."

The Power of Caregiving: Michael's Story

Michael, a devoted husband, became his wife's primary caregiver after her stroke. He learned new skills, from assisting with daily tasks to advocating for her medical needs. It was not always easy, but Michael found support groups and resources that helped him cope with the challenges. "Caregiving can be demanding," he admits, "but seeing my wife regain her independence makes it all worthwhile. We face this journey together, one step at a time."

Finding Hope After Loss: Emily's Story

Emily's father suffered a severe stroke, leaving him with long-term disabilities. Facing a future they hadn't planned, Emily and her family focused on creating a new normal. They adapted their home, embraced new routines, and celebrated small victories. "It was not the life we expected," Emily says, "but we found joy in the present. We learned to adapt and create new memories together."

The Importance of Community: John's Story

John, a stroke survivor, found solace and support in a stroke survivor support group. Sharing experiences, offering encouragement, and learning from each other created a sense of community. John says, "The group became my lifeline. I realized I was not alone. We all had challenges, but together, we found strength and hope."

Every Story is Unique, But Hope is Universal

These are just a few stories of the countless individuals touched by stroke. Each journey is unique, filled with its own challenges and triumphs. Yet, a common thread binds them all: hope, resilience, and the unwavering support of loved ones and communities.

Remember:

- **Recovery is a Journey:** There will be setbacks and victories. Celebrate your progress, no matter how small.
- **You Are Not Alone:** A vast community of stroke survivors and caregivers understand your challenges and offer support.
- **Hope is Always Possible:** With determination, support, and a positive attitude, you can rebuild your life after stroke.

Finding Inspiration and Strength in Shared Experiences

The stories in this chapter offer a glimpse into the remarkable strength and resilience of stroke survivors and caregivers. By learning from their experiences, you can find encouragement and hope on your own recovery journey. Remember, you are surrounded by a supportive community, and with a positive outlook, you can overcome challenges and build a fulfilling life after stroke.

Stroke Advocacy and Raising Awareness

Imagine a world where stroke prevention is prioritized, and stroke survivors have access to the best possible care and support. Stroke advocacy and raising awareness are crucial steps towards making this vision a reality. This chapter empowers you to become an advocate for yourself and others impacted by stroke.

Why is Stroke Advocacy Important?

Stroke is a leading cause of disability and death worldwide. Here is why advocacy matters:

- **Increased Funding for Research:** Advocacy can lead to more funding for research into stroke prevention, treatment, and recovery.
- **Improved Healthcare Policies:** Advocates can push for better policies that ensure stroke survivors have access to quality care and rehabilitation.
- **Public Awareness:** Raising awareness educates people about stroke risk factors, symptoms, and the importance of seeking immediate medical attention.
- **Empowering Stroke Survivors:** Advocacy allows stroke survivors to have a voice in shaping their healthcare experience and future.

How Can You Become a Stroke Advocate?

Here are some ways you can get involved in stroke advocacy:

- **Share Your Story:** Personal stories can be powerful tools for raising awareness. Talk to friends, family, or community groups about your experience.
- **Support Advocacy Organizations:** Donate your time, money, or voice to organizations fighting for stroke awareness and better care.
- **Educate Yourself:** Learn about stroke risk factors, prevention strategies, and available resources. Share this knowledge with others.
- **Connect with Legislators:** Contact your local representatives and urge them to support legislation that benefits stroke survivors.
- **Organize Events:** Host fundraising walks, awareness campaigns, or educational workshops in your community.

The Power of Small Actions

Even small actions can make a big difference in stroke advocacy. Here are some simple things you can do:

- **Wear Red for Stroke Awareness Day:** Participating in awareness campaigns sends a powerful message.
- **Talk to Your Doctor:** Discuss your stroke risk factors and ways to reduce them.
- **Spread Awareness on Social Media:** Share information about stroke prevention and resources online.

Remember:

- **Your Voice Matters:** You have the power to make a difference in the lives of others impacted by stroke.
- **Every Action Counts:** No contribution is too small when it comes to advocating for change.

- **Together We Can Make a Difference:** By joining forces, we can create a future where stroke is prevented, treated effectively, and survivors have the support they need.

Becoming a Stroke Advocate is a Rewarding Journey

Stroke advocacy empowers you to make a positive impact on a global issue. By sharing your story, raising awareness, and advocating for change, you can help create a brighter future for stroke survivors everywhere. Remember, your voice has the power to inspire and influence others. Become a champion for stroke awareness and make a difference in the world.

Cultural and Religious Considerations in Stroke Care

Imagine recovering from a stroke. You might wonder how your cultural or religious beliefs fit into your healthcare journey. This chapter explores the importance of considering cultural and religious beliefs in stroke care, ensuring your recovery process respects your values and traditions.

Understanding Cultural Diversity in Healthcare

People from different cultures have diverse beliefs about health, illness, and treatment. Here is what it means for stroke care:

- **Explaining Diagnosis and Treatment:** Healthcare providers should explain diagnoses and treatment options in a culturally sensitive way, respecting beliefs about illness and preferred communication styles.
- **Involving Family in Decision-Making:** Some cultures emphasize family involvement in medical decisions. Healthcare providers should recognize this and include family members appropriately.

- **Spiritual Practices and Healing:** Some cultures incorporate religious rituals or traditional healers into their healthcare practices. Respecting these practices can enhance recovery.

Respecting Religious Beliefs

Religious beliefs can also play a role in stroke care. Here are some considerations:

- **Dietary Restrictions:** Religious dietary restrictions should be accommodated during hospitalization and rehabilitation.
- **Prayer and Religious Practices:** Patients should be allowed to practice their faith freely, including prayer, visits from religious leaders, or observing religious holidays.
- **End-of-Life Care:** Religious beliefs might influence preferences for end-of-life care. Discuss your wishes openly with healthcare providers and loved ones.

Effective Communication is Key

Open communication is crucial to ensuring culturally and religiously sensitive care. Here are some tips:

- **Inform Your Doctor:** Share your cultural and religious background with your healthcare providers.
- **Ask Questions:** Do not hesitate to ask questions about how treatment aligns with your beliefs.
- **Seek Support:** Social workers or chaplains can help bridge the gap between your beliefs and healthcare practices.

Finding a Balance Between Cultures

Sometimes, cultural beliefs might differ from medical recommendations. Here is how to navigate these situations:

- **Open Dialogue:** Discuss any concerns with your doctor. They can explain the medical reasoning behind recommendations while respecting your beliefs.
- **Finding Common Ground:** There might be ways to modify treatment plans or incorporate aspects of your cultural or religious practices to achieve optimal outcomes.
- **Respecting Your Decisions:** Ultimately, the decision on your care lies with you. Healthcare providers should respect your informed choices.

Remember:

- **You Have Rights:** You have the right to culturally and religiously sensitive care that respects your values and beliefs.
- **Communication is Key:** Open communication with healthcare providers ensures your needs and wishes are understood.
- **Together We Can Find Solutions:** Healthcare providers can work with you to find a care plan that considers both medical best practices and your cultural or religious beliefs.

A Holistic Approach to Stroke Care

Cultural and religious beliefs are an essential part of who you are. Incorporating these beliefs into your stroke care plan fosters a more holistic healing process. By fostering open communication and respecting your traditions, healthcare providers can deliver care that aligns with your values and optimizes your recovery journey.

Remember, you are not alone. Healthcare providers are there to support your recovery while respecting your unique cultural and religious background.

9. SUPPORT FOR CAREGIVERS

Self-Care for Stroke Caregivers

Imagine being a superhero for your loved one after a stroke. You are there for every therapy session, helping with daily tasks, and offering emotional support. But what about you? Caregiving can be demanding, and neglecting your own well-being can lead to burnout. This chapter highlights the importance of self-care for stroke caregivers, offering tips and strategies to help you recharge and become the best version of yourself for your loved one.

Why is Self-Care Important for Caregivers?

Self-care is not selfish; it is essential. Here is why:

- **Prevents Burnout:** Taking care of yourself prevents exhaustion and allows you to offer better care for your loved one in the long run.
- **Reduces Stress:** Self-care activities help manage stress, which can improve your physical and mental health.
- **Boosts Emotional Well-being:** Taking care of yourself allows you to maintain a positive outlook and better cope with challenges.
- **Sets a Good Example:** By prioritizing self-care, you show your loved one the importance of taking care of their own well-being.

Simple Strategies for Self-Care

Self-care can be as simple as taking a few minutes for yourself each day. Here are some ideas:

- **Physical Activity:** Regular exercise, even a brisk walk, improves mood, reduces stress, and boosts energy levels.

- **Healthy Eating:** Nourish your body with nutritious meals and snacks to stay energized and focused.
- **Relaxation Techniques:** Practice deep breathing, meditation, or yoga to manage stress and promote relaxation.
- **Get Enough Sleep:** Aim for 7-8 hours of quality sleep each night to recharge your mind and body.
- **Connect with Others:** Schedule time for social activities with friends, family, or support groups for caregivers.
- **Do Something You Enjoy:** Make time for hobbies, reading, or activities that bring you joy and a sense of accomplishment.

Finding Time for Self-Care

Caregiving can be time-consuming, but self-care is not a luxury; it is a necessity. Here are some tips for carving out "me-time":

- **Delegate Tasks:** Ask family members, friends, or community services to help with some caregiving responsibilities.
- **Schedule Self-Care:** Treat self-care activities like important appointments and stick to the schedule.
- **Start Small:** Even small breaks can make a difference. Begin with 15 minutes a day for yourself and gradually increase the time.
- **Communicate Your Needs:** Let your loved one and family know you need time for self-care and explain its importance.

Remember:

- **You Are Not Alone:** Many people juggle caregiving responsibilities. There are resources and support groups available.
- **Taking Care of Yourself Is not Selfish:** It allows you to be a better caregiver for your loved one.
- **Small Steps Make a Big Difference:** Start with simple self-care practices and gradually build a routine that works for you.

Self-Care: The Foundation of Successful Caregiving

Prioritizing self-care empowers you to provide the best possible care for your loved one. By taking care of your physical, mental, and emotional well-being, you will have the energy, resilience, and positive attitude needed to navigate this journey. Remember, a well-rested and healthy caregiver is a more effective caregiver. Embrace self-care as a vital part of your caregiving journey, and watch your well-being and your loved one's recovery flourish.

Support Groups and Respite Care for Caregivers

Imagine caring for a loved one after a stroke. You might feel overwhelmed, isolated, and in need of support. This chapter explores two lifelines for caregivers: support groups and respite care. Here, you will discover how these resources can help you navigate your caregiving journey with greater confidence and peace of mind.

The Power of Support Groups

Support groups connect you with others who understand the challenges and rewards of caregiving. Here is how they can benefit you:

- **Shared Experiences:** Talking to people who "get it" can alleviate feelings of isolation and validate your emotions.
- **Practical Advice:** Learn valuable tips and strategies from other caregivers on managing daily tasks and navigating medical care.
- **Emotional Support:** Find encouragement, understanding, and a shoulder to lean on during difficult times.
- **Building Connections:** Develop friendships with others who share your journey, fostering a sense of community.

Finding the Right Support Group

Here are some tips for finding a support group that fits your needs:

- **Ask Your Doctor:** They might be aware of stroke caregiver support groups in your area.
- **Search Online:** Look for local support groups through stroke organizations or online forums.
- **Consider Your Preferences:** Choose a group that meets in person or online, depending on your comfort level. Some groups cater to specific needs, like caregivers of stroke survivors with aphasia.

Respite Care: A Well-Deserved Break

Respite care provides temporary relief from your caregiving responsibilities. This allows you to recharge and return to your role with renewed energy. Here are some types of respite care:

- **In-Home Care:** A qualified caregiver comes to your home to provide assistance while you take a break.
- **Adult Day Care Centers:** Your loved one spends the day in a safe and stimulating environment, participating in activities while you have time for yourself.
- **Short-Term Stays in Nursing Homes:** Your loved one receives temporary care in a nursing home, allowing you to take a longer break, such as a vacation.

Exploring Respite Care Options

Here are some things to consider when choosing respite care:

- **Your Loved One's Needs:** Ensure the care provider can meet your loved one's physical and emotional needs.
- **Your Budget:** Respite care can vary in cost. Explore options like insurance coverage or financial assistance programs.
- **Your Preferences:** Choose a respite care setting that aligns with your comfort level and budget.

Remember:

- **You Do not Have to Go It Alone:** Support groups connect you with others who understand your challenges.
- **Respite Care Is not a Sign of Weakness:** It is a sign of a responsible caregiver prioritizing their well-being.
- **Help is Available:** There are resources and support systems to help you navigate the caregiving journey.

Finding Strength in Numbers and Taking Time for Yourself

Support groups and respite care are essential resources for stroke caregivers. Sharing your journey with others who understand provides emotional support and valuable advice. Respite care allows you to take a break and recharge, ensuring you can continue caring for your loved one with renewed energy and a positive attitude. Remember, seeking support and taking care of yourself are not signs of weakness; they are essential steps in becoming a stronger and more effective caregiver on this journey. Embrace these resources, find solace in shared experiences, and allow yourself the time to breathe. You are not alone.

Managing Stress and Avoiding Burnout

Imagine dedicating yourself to caring for a loved one after a stroke. The constant demands can leave you feeling stressed, exhausted, and on the verge of burnout. This chapter equips you with essential tools to manage stress and prevent burnout, ensuring you can provide the best care for yourself and your loved one.

Understanding Caregiver Stress

Caregiving can be incredibly rewarding, but it also comes with significant challenges. Here is why stress is common:

- **Constant Demands:** Caregiving often involves long hours, physical exertion, and emotional strain.
- **Uncertainties and Challenges:** Navigating medical care, dealing with behavioral changes, and facing the unknown can be overwhelming.
- **Feeling Overwhelmed:** Juggling caregiving responsibilities with your own work, family, and personal life can lead to feeling stretched too thin.
- **Isolation and Loneliness:** Focusing on your loved one's needs can leave you feeling isolated and unable to confide in others.

Recognizing the Signs of Burnout

Burnout is a state of emotional, physical, and mental exhaustion. Here are some warning signs:

- **Constant Fatigue:** You feel drained and exhausted, even after getting enough sleep.
- **Increased Cynicism:** You might feel detached or negative towards your caregiving role.
- **Decreased Sense of Accomplishment:** You feel like your efforts do not make a difference, leading to a loss of motivation.
- **Changes in Eating and Sleeping Habits:** You might experience unhealthy eating habits or difficulty sleeping.
- **Withdrawing from Social Activities:** You lose interest in activities you once enjoyed and isolate yourself from others.

Strategies for Managing Stress

Here are some practical tips for managing stress and preventing burnout:

- **Prioritize Self-Care:** Schedule time for activities you enjoy, like exercise, relaxation techniques, or spending time with loved ones.

- **Set Realistic Expectations:** Accept that you cannot control everything. Focus on what you can do and delegate tasks whenever possible.
- **Ask for Help:** Do not be afraid to reach out to family, friends, or respite care services for support.
- **Join a Support Group:** Connecting with others who understand your challenges can be incredibly helpful.
- **Communicate Effectively:** Talk openly with your loved one and healthcare providers about your concerns and needs.
- **Practice Relaxation Techniques:** Deep breathing, meditation, or yoga can help manage stress and promote relaxation.

Remember:

- **Taking Care of Yourself Is not Selfish:** A well-rested and healthy caregiver is a more effective caregiver.
- **You Are Not Alone:** Many people experience caregiver stress. There are resources and support systems available.
- **Stress Management is a Continuous Process:** Develop healthy coping mechanisms and make self-care a regular part of your routine.

Building Resilience and Avoiding Burnout

By actively managing stress and prioritizing your well-being, you can build resilience and avoid burnout. Remember, you are on a marathon, not a sprint. By taking care of yourself and utilizing available resources, you can approach your caregiving journey with a sense of calm, confidence, and renewed energy. You are doing an amazing job, and do not forget to take care of yourself along the way.

Legal and Financial Considerations for Caregivers

Imagine yourself caring for a loved one after a stroke. While love and dedication are essential, legal and financial considerations arise. This chapter explores crucial aspects of planning for the future, ensuring you can best support your loved one while protecting your own well-being.

Understanding Your Legal Responsibilities

Caregiving often involves making decisions on your loved one's behalf. Here is what you need to know:

- **Power of Attorney:** This legal document allows you to make medical and financial decisions if your loved one becomes incapacitated. Discuss their wishes and ensure this document is up-to-date.
- **Guardianship:** In some cases, legal guardianship might be necessary, granting you legal authority over your loved one's personal and financial decisions.
- **Advance Directives:** These documents outline your loved one's wishes for end-of-life care, ensuring their preferences are respected.

Planning for Financial Burdens

Stroke care can be expensive. Here are some things to consider:

- **Medical Bills:** Explore insurance coverage, government assistance programs, and payment plans to manage healthcare costs.
- **Long-Term Care Expenses:** If long-term care facilities are needed, research your options, and explore financial assistance programs.
- **Impact on Your Finances:** Caregiving might affect your work schedule. Explore benefits like FMLA (Family and Medical Leave Act) and consider financial planning strategies.

Navigating Legal and Financial Decisions

Here are some tips for navigating legal and financial considerations:

- **Seek Legal Advice:** Consult an attorney specializing in elder law to understand your legal responsibilities and options.
- **Communicate with Your Loved One:** Discuss their wishes for care and finances while they are still able to make decisions.
- **Gather Important Documents:** Organize medical records, insurance information, and financial documents for easy access.
- **Explore Financial Resources:** Research government benefits, veteran's benefits, or disability programs that might offer financial assistance.

Remember:

- **Planning Ahead is Key:** Early planning allows you to make informed decisions and avoid unnecessary stress during a difficult time.
- **Knowledge is Power:** Educate yourself about legal and financial aspects of caregiving to make informed choices.
- **Seek Professional Help:** Do not hesitate to seek legal and financial guidance from qualified professionals.

Making Informed Choices for a Secure Future

By understanding your legal responsibilities and planning for potential financial burdens, you can ensure your loved one receives the best possible care while protecting your own well-being. Remember, planning ahead does not take away from the present; it empowers you to navigate challenges stnd focus on what matters most – caring for your loved one. With knowledge, resources, and guidance, you can approach the future with a sense of control and confidence.

Setting Boundaries and Saying No as a Caregiver

Imagine devoting yourself to caring for a loved one after a stroke. You want to be there for them, but the constant demands leave you feeling stretched thin. This chapter explores the importance of setting boundaries and saying no as a caregiver. By prioritizing self-care and establishing healthy limits, you can become a more effective caregiver in the long run.

Why Are Boundaries Important for Caregivers?

Caregiving can be rewarding, but it can also lead to resentment and burnout if boundaries are blurred. Here is why boundaries matter:

- **Preventing Caregiver Burnout:** Saying no to unreasonable requests allows you to manage your energy and avoid exhaustion.
- **Maintaining Your Relationships:** Time for friends, family, and hobbies helps you maintain balance and avoid social isolation.
- **Prioritizing Your Health:** Self-care activities like exercise and relaxation are crucial for your physical and mental well-being.
- **Setting a Healthy Example:** By setting boundaries, you show your loved one the importance of self-respect and self-care.

Learning to Say No Effectively

Saying no does not mean you do not care. Here are some tips for communicating boundaries effectively:

- **Be Clear and Direct:** State your refusal clearly and calmly. Explain why you cannot take on additional tasks.
- **Offer Alternatives:** Suggest alternative solutions or ways someone else might be able to help.
- **Focus on Your Needs:** Explain how saying no helps you care for yourself and ultimately care better for your loved one.

- **Use "I" Statements:** Instead of accusatory language, use phrases like "I need time for myself" or "I cannot manage this today."

Examples of Setting Boundaries

Here are some situations where setting boundaries might be necessary:

- **Saying No to Unrealistic Demands:** If someone expects you to be available 24/7, explain your need for breaks and downtime.
- **Limiting Social Activities:** It is okay to decline invitations if you need time for yourself or your loved one.
- **Delegating Tasks:** Do not be afraid to ask family, friends, or professional services for help with some caregiving tasks.

Remember:

- **You Have the Right to Say No:** Setting boundaries is a healthy way to manage your caregiving responsibilities.
- **Guilt Does not Help:** Taking care of yourself is not selfish; it makes you a better caregiver.
- **Communication is Key:** Explain your boundaries clearly and calmly to avoid misunderstandings.

Creating a Sustainable Caregiving Journey

Setting boundaries is not about abandoning your loved one; it is about creating a sustainable caregiving journey. By prioritizing self-care and establishing healthy limits, you can manage your energy, maintain your well-being, and ultimately become a more effective caregiver for your loved one. Remember, a healthy and balanced caregiver is better equipped to provide the love and support your loved one needs. So, do not be afraid to say no, and prioritize your well-being. You deserve it, and your loved one deserves the best version of you.

10. PROFESSIONAL RESOURCES

A Guide for Healthcare Professionals Working with Stroke Survivors in the Home Setting

Imagine being a healthcare professional dedicated to helping stroke survivors recover in the comfort of their own homes. This chapter equips you with essential knowledge and strategies to optimize patient care in the home environment.

Understanding the Home Setting

Transitioning from hospital to home can be a significant adjustment for stroke survivors. Here is what to consider:

- **Individual Needs:** Each survivor has unique needs based on their stroke severity, limitations, and living situation.
- **Home Environment:** Assess the home for safety hazards, accessibility, and modifications needed to facilitate recovery.
- **Family and Caregiver Support:** Evaluate the support system available at home and identify areas where education or resources might be needed.

Optimizing Care in the Home

Here are key strategies for providing effective care in the home setting:

- **Goal Setting and Collaboration:** Work collaboratively with the stroke survivor and their family to establish realistic goals for rehabilitation.
- **Patient Education:** Empower the survivor and their caregivers with education on stroke recovery, medication management, and techniques for daily living activities.

- **Communication and Coordination:** Maintain clear communication with the survivor, family, and other healthcare providers involved in the care plan.
- **Monitoring Progress:** Regularly assess the survivor's progress towards goals, adjusting the care plan as needed.
- **Emotional and Social Support:** Recognize the emotional challenges of stroke recovery and offer support and resources for mental well-being.

Addressing Specific Challenges

Stroke survivors might face various challenges at home. Here is how to address some common ones:

- **Mobility Issues:** Provide guidance on safe mobility techniques, assistive devices, and potential home modifications.
- **Cognitive Difficulties:** Offer strategies for memory impairment, communication challenges, and problem-solving difficulties.
- **Speech and Language Impairments:** Connect the survivor with speech therapists to improve communication skills.
- **Emotional and Social Issues:** Address depression, anxiety, and social isolation by providing resources for mental health support and social connection.

Collaboration is Key

Effective home-based care relies on collaboration with various stakeholders:

- **The Stroke Survivor:** They are the central figure in their recovery journey. Active participation in goal setting and therapy is crucial.
- **Family and Caregivers:** Providing education and support empowers caregivers to offer the best possible assistance.

- **Other Healthcare Professionals:** Maintain communication with therapists, rehabilitation specialists, and social workers involved in the care plan.

Remember:

- **Individualized Care is Essential:** Tailor your approach to each survivor's unique needs and home environment.
- **Empowerment is Key:** Focus on equipping stroke survivors and caregivers with knowledge and skills to manage their recovery journey.
- **Partnership Leads to Success:** Collaboration among healthcare professionals, the survivor, and their support system optimizes recovery outcomes.

Building a Bridge to Recovery

Working with stroke survivors in their home environment can be a fulfilling experience. By understanding the unique challenges and strategies for providing effective care at home, you can become a valuable partner in their recovery journey. Remember, your expertise and guidance can empower stroke survivors to regain independence, improve their quality of life, and thrive in the comfort of their own homes.

Ethical Considerations in Home Care for Stroke Patients

Imagine yourself as a healthcare professional providing home care for a stroke survivor. You prioritize their well-being, but ethical dilemmas can arise. This chapter explores these complexities, equipping you to make informed decisions that uphold patient autonomy, safety, and best practices.

Balancing Patient Autonomy and Safety

Stroke survivors have the right to make choices about their care. However, their judgment might be impaired. Here is how to navigate this challenge:

- **Promoting Informed Consent:** Ensure the survivor understands treatment options, risks, and benefits, even if it requires multiple explanations in simple terms.
- **Respecting Choices, Even Difficult Ones:** If a survivor makes an informed decision you disagree with, discuss the risks and explore alternatives. Ultimately, respect their autonomy.
- **Involving Family (with Caution):** Family can be a valuable resource, but avoid pressuring the survivor into choices they do not want.

Confidentiality and Privacy in the Home Setting

Home care involves a more personal environment. Here is how to maintain confidentiality and privacy:

- **Limit Information Sharing:** Share patient information only with those directly involved in their care and with the survivor's consent.
- **Respect Privacy During Visits:** Minimize the number of healthcare professionals present during home visits and ensure a private space for discussions.
- **Be Mindful of Family Dynamics:** Maintain confidentiality even within families, especially if there are disagreements about care.

Allocation of Resources and Fair Treatment

Healthcare resources are not unlimited. Here is how to ensure fair treatment for stroke survivors receiving home care:

- **Advocate for Necessary Services:** Do not hesitate to advocate for essential therapies, equipment, or modifications the survivor needs, even if resources are limited.
- **Document Needs Clearly:** Maintain accurate documentation of the survivor's needs to justify the allocation of resources.
- **Be Aware of Implicit Bias:** Ensure all stroke survivors receive fair treatment regardless of background, socioeconomic status, or disability level.

Addressing End-of-Life Care at Home

Stroke can raise complex end-of-life considerations. Here is how to approach these sensitive situations:

- **Supporting Advance Directives:** Discuss advance directives with the survivor and family to ensure their wishes are respected regarding end-of-life care.
- **Providing Emotional Support:** Offer emotional support and resources to the survivor and their family as they navigate difficult decisions.
- **Collaboration with Hospice:** If appropriate, collaborate with hospice care providers to ensure comfort and dignity during the end stages of life.

Working as a Team: Ethical Decision-Making

Ethical dilemmas are often complex. Here is how to make informed decisions:

- **Seek Consultation:** Discuss ethical concerns with colleagues, supervisors, or ethics committees within your healthcare organization.
- **Document Your Reasoning:** Clearly document the ethical considerations, your thought process, and the final decision made.

- **Staying Up-to-Date:** Keep yourself informed about evolving ethical guidelines and best practices in home care for stroke patients.

Remember:

- **Open Communication is Key:** Maintain open and honest communication with the survivor, family, and other healthcare professionals involved.
- **Seek Guidance When Needed:** Do not hesitate to seek guidance from colleagues or ethics committees when facing complex ethical dilemmas.
- **Upholding Patient Rights:** Always prioritize the rights, safety, and well-being of the stroke survivor in your decision-making.

Building Trust Through Ethical Care

Home care for stroke survivors requires ethical considerations alongside clinical expertise. By prioritizing patient autonomy, advocating for their needs, and navigating ethical dilemmas with transparency, you can build trust and ensure the delivery of high-quality, compassionate care in the comfort of their own home. Remember, your ethical conduct plays a crucial role in optimizing the recovery journey for stroke survivors.

Educational Resources for Healthcare Professionals on Home Stroke Care

Imagine yourself as a healthcare professional dedicated to helping stroke survivors recover in their own homes. You possess the clinical skills, but keeping up-to-date on the latest advancements in home stroke care is essential. This chapter explores valuable educational resources to equip you with the knowledge and expertise to provide exceptional care in the home setting.

Why Continuous Learning is Important

The field of stroke care is constantly evolving. Here is why staying informed is crucial:

- **Improved Patient Outcomes:** Staying current on best practices in home stroke care allows you to deliver the most effective interventions for optimal patient recovery.
- **Enhanced Caregiver Education:** The latest knowledge empowers you to better educate caregivers on stroke recovery, fostering a collaborative approach to care.
- **Addressing Evolving Needs:** Stroke survivors may face new challenges throughout their recovery journey. Continuous learning equips you to address these evolving needs effectively.

Exploring Educational Resources

A wealth of educational resources is available for healthcare professionals working in home stroke care. Here are some key options:

- **Professional Organizations:** National and international stroke organizations like the American Stroke Association and the World Stroke Organization offer online courses, conferences, and educational materials on various aspects of home stroke care.
- **Online Learning Platforms:** Several online platforms offer accredited continuing education courses specifically designed for healthcare professionals working in stroke rehabilitation and home care.
- **Medical Journals and Publications:** Stay current with the latest research findings by subscribing to reputable medical journals specializing in stroke and rehabilitation medicine.
- **Webinars and Conferences:** Attend webinars and conferences hosted by stroke organizations or healthcare institutions to gain insights from leading experts in home stroke care.

Enhancing Your Skillset

Here are some specific areas where ongoing education can significantly benefit your practice:

- **Post-Stroke Rehabilitation Techniques:** Learn about the latest therapeutic approaches for improving mobility, communication, cognitive function, and activities of daily living (ADLs) in the home environment.
- **Home Modifications for Stroke Survivors:** Educate yourself on strategies for modifying homes to improve accessibility and safety for stroke survivors.
- **Communication Strategies for Stroke Survivors with Aphasia:** Develop effective communication techniques to support stroke survivors experiencing aphasia, a language disorder that can occur after a stroke.
- **Mental Health Considerations in Stroke Recovery:** Learn to identify and address potential mental health challenges like depression and anxiety that stroke survivors might face.

Building a Collaborative Learning Network

In addition to individual learning, consider these collaborative approaches:

- **Journal Clubs:** Form a journal club with colleagues to discuss and share recent research findings on home stroke care.
- **Mentorship Programs:** Seek mentorship from experienced healthcare professionals specializing in home stroke care.
- **Interdisciplinary Collaboration:** Participate in discussions and learning initiatives with other healthcare professionals involved in stroke care, such as therapists, social workers, and nurses.

Remember:

- **Lifelong Learning is Essential:** Continuous learning is crucial for staying current in the ever-evolving field of stroke care.
- **Diverse Resources are Available:** Explore a variety of educational resources to cater to your learning preferences and specific areas of interest.
- **Shared Knowledge Benefits Patients:** By actively seeking knowledge and collaborating with colleagues, you can elevate the quality of care provided to stroke survivors in the home setting.

Investing in Your Expertise Empowers Stroke Recovery

Healthcare professionals play a vital role in optimizing stroke recovery in the home environment. By dedicating yourself to continuous learning and staying abreast of the latest advancements in home stroke care, you can ensure you deliver the most effective interventions and empower stroke survivors to achieve their full recovery potential. Remember, your commitment to lifelong learning paves the way for a brighter future for stroke survivors returning home.

Building a Care Team for Stroke Survivors in the Home Setting

Imagine being discharged from the hospital after a stroke. You might feel a mix of relief and anxiety about recovery at home. This chapter explores the importance of building a care team, your personal A-Team, to support you on this journey.

Why is a Care Team Important in-Home Care?

Stroke recovery is a complex process with various needs. Here is why a care team is essential:

- **Comprehensive Care:** A team approach ensures you receive the full spectrum of support needed for physical, mental, and emotional well-being.
- **Specialized Expertise:** Each team member brings their unique expertise to address specific aspects of your recovery, like physical therapy, speech therapy, or social work.
- **Continuity of Care:** The team works together to create a coordinated care plan, ensuring smooth transitions between different healthcare providers.

Who Makes Up Your Home Care Team?

The specific members of your care team will vary based on your individual needs. Here are some key players:

- **Physician:** Your primary care doctor or a neurologist oversees your overall health and medication management.
- **Rehabilitation Team:** This might include physical therapists, occupational therapists, and speech-language pathologists who help you regain mobility, communication skills, and daily living skills.
- **Home Health Nurse:** A nurse can provide skilled care at home, monitor your health, and educate you and your caregivers.
- **Social Worker:** Social workers can connect you with community resources, assist with financial planning, and offer emotional support.
- **Mental Health Professionals:** A psychologist or therapist can address anxiety, depression, or other mental health challenges that might arise after stroke.
- **Caregivers:** Your family members or hired caregivers provide daily assistance with tasks like bathing, dressing, and meal preparation.

Building a Team that Works for You

Here are some tips for building an effective care team:

- **Communicate with Your Doctor:** Discuss your needs and preferences with your doctor. They can recommend qualified team members.
- **Ask Questions:** Do not hesitate to ask questions about each team member's role and qualifications.
- **Consider Your Preferences:** Choose team members who you feel comfortable with and who communicate effectively.
- **Focus on Collaboration:** Encourage open communication and collaboration among team members to ensure a unified care plan.

Remember:

- **You Are in Charge:** You have the right to choose the members of your care team and have a say in your care plan.
- **Communication is Key:** Open communication between team members and with you is vital for a successful recovery journey.
- **The Right Team Empowers Recovery:** A well-coordinated care team provides the comprehensive support and expertise you need to thrive at home after a stroke.

Building a Support System for a Brighter Future

A care team is not just about medical professionals; it is your support system during and beyond recovery. By collaborating with a team of qualified and compassionate individuals, you can feel confident and empowered on your journey back to a fulfilling life at home. Remember, you are not alone. With the right team by your side, you can overcome challenges and achieve your full recovery potential.

11. ADDITIONAL TOPICS

Children and Stroke: A Caregiver's Guide

Imagine the world turned upside down. Your child, full of energy and curiosity, is suddenly facing a medical challenge – a stroke. This chapter is here to support you, the caregiver, on this unexpected journey. Here, you will find information and resources to help your child heal and your family cope.

Understanding Childhood Stroke

Strokes can happen at any age, including children. Here is what you need to know:

- **Types of Childhood Stroke:** Strokes in children can be caused by blood clots, bleeding in the brain, or problems with blood vessel formation.
- **Symptoms:** Signs of stroke in children can vary, but may include weakness or numbness on one side of the body, slurred speech, facial drooping, or sudden seizures.
- **Importance of Early Action:** Early diagnosis and treatment are crucial for minimizing long-term effects. If you suspect a stroke, seek immediate medical attention.

Supporting Your Child's Recovery

The recovery process for a child after a stroke can be long and require patience. Here are some ways you can support your child:

- **Follow Treatment Plans:** Work closely with healthcare professionals to understand and diligently follow their recommendations for therapy, medication, and rehabilitation.

- **Focus on Communication:** Children might struggle with communication after a stroke. Be patient and practice communication techniques recommended by therapists.
- **Maintain a Positive Environment:** Create a loving and supportive home environment that encourages healing and celebrates small victories.
- **Connect with Others:** Seek support groups or connect with families who have been through similar experiences. Sharing can be a source of strength.

Addressing Emotional Challenges

A stroke can be a frightening experience for a child. Here is how to address their emotional well-being:

- **Open Communication:** Encourage your child to express their feelings and answer their questions honestly and in a way they can understand.
- **Age-Appropriate Explanations:** Explain the situation in a simple way, tailored to your child's age and understanding.
- **Emotional Support:** Offer reassurance, love, and support. Let them know you are there for them every step of the way.
- **Consider Therapy:** If your child is struggling emotionally, explore child therapy options to help them cope with the changes and challenges they face.

Helping Siblings Adjust

A child's stroke can affect the whole family. Here are some tips to help siblings adjust:

- **Honest Communication:** Talk to your other children about what happened and answer their questions honestly.

- **Reassure Their Well-being:** Let them know they are loved and safe.
- **Acknowledge Their Feelings:** They might feel scared, confused, or even resentful. Listen to their concerns and validate their emotions.
- **Maintain Normalcy:** As much as possible, maintain routines and traditions to provide a sense of normalcy for your other children.

Remember:

- **You Are Not Alone:** There are resources and support groups available for families dealing with childhood stroke.
- **Early Intervention is Key:** Early diagnosis and treatment can significantly improve your child's recovery outcomes.
- **Focus on Love and Support:** Your love and unwavering support are essential for your child's healing journey.

A Journey of Hope and Resilience

Childhood stroke can be a difficult experience, but with knowledge, support, and the right care plan, your child can make significant progress. This chapter equips you with the tools to navigate this journey. Remember, you are a strong advocate for your child. Do not hesitate to ask questions, seek help, and stay positive. Together, you can help your child heal and build a brighter future.

Stroke and Technology

Imagine yourself recovering from a stroke. Regaining mobility, communication, and independence can feel like a daunting task. This chapter dives into the exciting world of technology like apps, devices, and online resources designed to empower your stroke recovery journey.

How Technology Can Assist Stroke Recovery

Technology offers a multitude of tools to enhance your rehabilitation and daily life:

- **Exercise and Therapy Apps:** Interactive apps can guide you through physical and cognitive exercises, making therapy more engaging and accessible.
- **Communication Aids:** Speech-generating apps and other assistive technologies can help overcome communication challenges caused by stroke.
- **Medication Management Apps:** Apps can remind you to take medication, track progress, and even connect you with pharmacists for questions.
- **Assistive Devices for Daily Living:** Smart home devices can control lights, thermostats, and appliances with voice commands or modified interfaces, increasing independence.
- **Educational Resources:** Websites and online communities offer reliable information on stroke recovery, support groups, and inspirational stories.

Exploring Useful Apps

Here are some examples of helpful apps to consider:

- **Exercise Apps:** Look for apps with customizable exercises for physical and cognitive rehabilitation, some focusing on balance, coordination, or memory improvement.
- **Communication Apps:** Explore apps that offer text-to-speech conversion, picture symbols, or word prediction features to aid communication.
- **Medication Management Apps:** Choose apps with features like dosage reminders, refill alerts, and medication interaction checkers.

Finding the Right Tech for You

With so many options, choosing the right technology can be overwhelming. Here are some tips:

- **Consider Your Needs:** Identify your specific recovery goals and daily living challenges.
- **Seek Recommendations:** Talk to your doctor, therapist, or rehabilitation counselor for suggestions.
- **Read Reviews and Ratings:** Research apps and devices online to find user reviews and ratings.
- **Try Before You Buy:** Many apps offer free trials, so you can test them out before committing.

Beyond Apps: Assistive Devices and Online Resources

Technology offers more than just apps. Here are some additional resources to explore:

- **Assistive Devices:** Consider voice-activated speakers, smart plugs for appliances, or adaptive utensils to simplify daily tasks.
- **Online Support Groups:** Connect with stroke survivors and caregivers online for peer support and shared experiences.
- **Educational Websites:** Trustworthy websites like the American Stroke Association offer reliable information on stroke recovery and prevention.

Remember:

- **Technology is a Tool:** Tech can be a valuable companion, but it shouldn't replace traditional therapy or professional guidance.
- **Focus on Accessibility:** Choose user-friendly apps and devices with clear interfaces and features that adapt to your abilities.

- **Embrace Continuous Learning:** The world of technology is constantly evolving. Explore new apps and resources as your needs change.

Building a Tech-Powered Recovery Journey

Technology is no magic bullet, but it can be a powerful ally in your stroke recovery journey. By using apps, devices, and online resources strategically, you can enhance your therapy, improve communication, manage daily tasks, and stay connected. Remember, technology empowers you to take an active role in your recovery and build a brighter future. So, explore what's out there, embrace innovation, and let technology be your partner on the path to a fulfilling life.

Traveling After Stroke

Imagine the world beckoning again. After a stroke, the thought of traveling might seem daunting. This chapter equips you, the stroke survivor, with essential tips and considerations to ensure safe and enjoyable adventures.

Planning for a Smooth Journey

Preparation is key to a stress-free travel experience:

- **Consult Your Doctor:** Discuss your travel plans with your doctor to ensure your health is stable and you are cleared for travel.
- **Gather Medical Documents:** Carry copies of your medical history, medications, and doctor's contact information in case of emergencies.
- **Consider Travel Insurance:** Explore travel insurance options that cover medical emergencies abroad.

- **Research Accessibility:** Choose destinations and accommodations that are accessible for your current mobility limitations.
- **Pack Smart:** Pack comfortable clothing, medications, and any necessary medical equipment. Consider packing a small first-aid kit as well.

Travel Considerations Based on Your Recovery

Here are some things to keep in mind depending on your recovery stage:

- **Early Recovery:** If you are still in early recovery, focus on short trips closer to home to rebuild confidence and stamina.
- **Limited Mobility:** Plan for destinations with accessible transportation, hotels with elevators and grab bars, and manageable walking distances.
- **Communication Challenges:** If you have difficulty speaking, consider traveling with a companion or learning basic phrases in the local language.

Travel Tips for a Safe and Enjoyable Experience

Here are some practical tips to make your travels more comfortable:

- **Pace Yourself:** Plan itineraries that allow for rest breaks and avoid overexertion.
- **Stay Hydrated:** Drink plenty of fluids, especially during travel and in hot climates.
- **Maintain Healthy Habits:** Continue your regular medication schedule and healthy eating habits as much as possible.
- **Pack Light:** Limit your luggage to avoid heavy lifting and potential strain.

- **Embrace Assistance:** Do not hesitate to ask for help from airport staff, airline personnel, or hotel employees.
- **Travel with a Companion:** Consider traveling with a friend or family member for added support and peace of mind.

Traveling with a Positive Attitude

A positive attitude is essential for a fulfilling travel experience:

- **Focus on Ability:** Focus on what you can do, not your limitations. There is still a world of adventure waiting to be explored.
- **Be Flexible:** Be prepared to adjust your plans or itinerary if needed.
- **Embrace New Experiences:** See travel as a chance to learn new things and create lasting memories.

Remember:

- Traveling After Stroke is Possible: With careful planning and the right precautions, you can still enjoy the joys of travel after a stroke.
- Your Health Comes First: Always prioritize your health and well-being when planning a trip.
- Embrace the Adventure: Travel can be a rewarding experience that fosters independence and a renewed zest for life. So, pack your bags, embrace the adventure, and get ready to explore the world again.

Stroke and Pets

Imagine this: you are now the primary caregiver for a loved one recovering from a stroke. While their health is your top priority, there is another furry friend to consider – your pet. This chapter explores how to manage pet care alongside the demands of stroke recovery, ensuring both your loved one and your pet receive the love and attention they need.

The Importance of Pets in Stroke Recovery

Pets can play a significant role in stroke recovery, offering:

- **Companionship:** Pets can provide emotional support and reduce feelings of loneliness, which are common after a stroke.
- **Motivation:** Walking or playing with a pet can encourage physical activity, crucial for stroke rehabilitation.
- **Stress Relief:** Caring for a pet can be calming and reduce stress levels for both the caregiver and the stroke survivor.

Challenges of Managing Pets During Stroke Recovery

However, caring for a pet can add another layer of responsibility:
- **Mobility Issues:** If your loved one's mobility is limited, walking, feeding, and cleaning up after a pet might become difficult.
- **Changes in Behavior:** A stroke can affect a person's behavior and ability to care for their pet. They might be less patient or energetic.
- **New Routines:** Changes in daily routines due to stroke recovery can disrupt pet schedules and cause anxiety.

Finding Solutions: Balancing Needs

Here is how to ensure your loved one, your pet, and yourself receive the care you all need:

- **Seek Help with Pet Care:** Consider asking family, friends, or pet-sitting services for help with walking, feeding, and cleaning up after your pet.
- **Maintain Routines (as much as possible):** Try to stick to your pet's regular feeding, walking, and playtime schedules to minimize disruption.

- **Adapt Activities:** If your loved one can no longer walk the dog, explore shorter walks or indoor playtime options.
- **Consider In-Home Rehabilitation:** Inquire about therapists who can incorporate pet interaction into rehabilitation exercises, promoting both physical and emotional well-being.
- **Identify Signs of Pet Stress:** Watch for changes in your pet's behavior, such as excessive barking, hiding, or loss of appetite, which might indicate stress due to the new situation. Address these concerns with a veterinarian or animal behaviorist.

Additional Tips for a Smooth Transition

Here are some additional ideas to make things easier:

- **Prepare a Pet Care Kit:** Create a kit with detailed pet care instructions, including feeding schedule, medication information, and emergency contact details for pet sitters or veterinarians.
- **Identify Pet-Friendly Resources:** Research local pet-friendly transportation options, dog parks, or doggy daycare facilities if needed.
- **Involve Your Loved One in Pet Care (if possible):** Even if your loved one's mobility is limited, encourage them to interact with the pet through petting, talking, or offering treats. This can provide comfort and a sense of purpose.

Remember:

- **Pets Can Be Part of the Recovery Journey:** Pets offer valuable companionship and support during stroke recovery.
- **Planning and Support are Key:** Planning ahead and seeking help with pet care can ensure the well-being of both your loved one and your furry companion.

- **Open Communication is Essential:** Talk to your veterinarian or animal behaviorist if you have concerns about your pet's adjustment or need advice on adapting pet care routines.

By taking these steps, you can ensure that both your loved one and your pet feel loved, supported, and cared for during this challenging time. Remember, with a little planning and creativity, you can create a harmonious environment where everyone thrives.

Can You Help Others Find This Book by Writing a Review?

Thank you for reading the book. As a retired physician with a fresh viewpoint, I am dedicating my time to creating this informative series out of a desire to empower others through credible information. This series is my way of continuing to serve others, not for profit, but out of a deep love and passion for sharing knowledge to benefit those who are perplexed by the overwhelming information overload in the digital world. Therefore, I have created this series of patient information books as a one-stop information haven, painstakingly built to save you valuable time. Your honest review on Amazon, accessible through the QR code below, will be a guiding light for others seeking clarity. Let us empower each other, one informed reader at a time! Kindly write a review about this book!

ABOUT THE AUTHOR

Dr. A. Mitra is a retired medical doctor who has worked in the field of General Practice in Family Medicine in India and Australia for over 30 years. He completed his graduate education in India and then did further studies in Australia and UK. Currently he lives a private modest life and pursues his interests in reading and writing on various topics.